Neuroscience Nursing

Scope and Standards of Practice

4th Edition

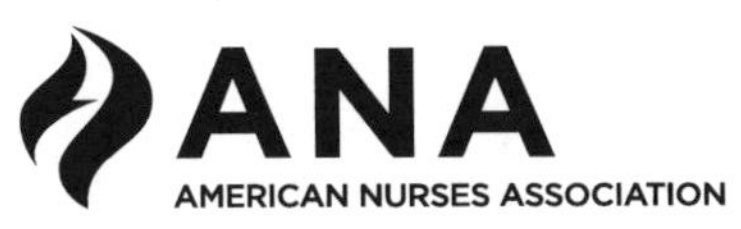

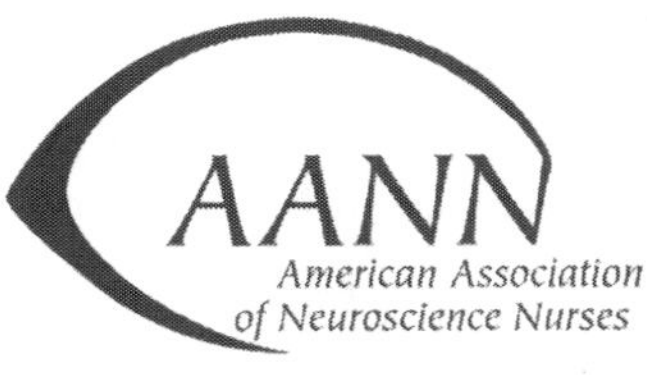

The American Nurses Association (ANA) and American Association of Neuroscience Nurses (AANN) are national professional associations. This publication reflects the position of the ANA and AANN regarding the scope and standards of nursing practice and should be reviewed in conjunction with state board of nursing regulations. State law, rules, and regulations govern the practice of nursing, while *Neuroscience Nursing: Scope and Standards of Practice* guides registered nurses in the application of their professional skills and responsibilities.

About the American Nurses Association
The ANA is the only full-service professional organization representing the interests of the nation's 4.2 million registered nurses through its constituent/state nurses associations and its organizational affiliates. The ANA advances the nursing profession by fostering high standards of nursing practice, promoting the rights of nurses in the workplace, projecting a positive and realistic view of nursing, and by lobbying the Congress and regulatory agencies on healthcare issues affecting nurses and the public.

About the American Association of Neuroscience Nurses
The AANN supports neuroscience nurses and their patients by providing continuing education and certification preparatory materials, disseminating information, setting standards, and advocating on behalf of neuroscience patients, families, and nurses. A neuroscience nurse is a nursing professional that helps patients with neurological disorders. This can include injuries, such as head and spinal trauma from accidents, or illnesses, such as Parkinson's disease, meningitis, encephalitis, epilepsy, and multiple sclerosis.

American Nurses Association
8515 Georgia Avenue, Suite 400
Silver Spring, MD 20910

Cataloging-in-Publication data on file with Library of Congress

ISBNs
Print 978-1-963052-07-7
ePDF 978-1-963052-08-4
ePUB 978-1-963052-09-1
Mobi 978-1-963052-10-7
SAN: 851-3481

Contents

Contributors

TASK FORCE

Janice L. Hinkle, PhD, RN, CNRN Task Force Co-Chairperson
Bethany C. Young, PhD, RN, AGCNS-BC, CCRN
Jessica Adame, MSN-Ed, RN, SCRN, CNRN
Nnedinma Agu, RN, BSN
Sarah Andrews, DNP, APRN, ACNS-BC, ANVP-BC, ASC, CRRN,
    SCRN, PCCN-K, CMSRN
Susan Bell, DNP, MS, RN, CNRN, APRN-CNP
Teresa Connolly, PhD, RN, ACNS-BC, CNRN
Laura Crawford, MSN, RN, CCRN-K, CNRN
Angel Duzan, DNP, RN, ACCNS-AG, CCRN-K, CNRN, SCRN
Susan D. Fuhrman, MS, RN, MSN, RN-BC, CCNS, APNP, FAHA
Lori Kennedy, PhD, RN, ACNP-BC, CCRN, CNRN, FNCS
Youngjin Kwon, MSN, RN, SCRN, CCRN
Minna B. Masor, EdD, MSN, RN, CCRN, SCRN
Malissa Mulkey, PhD, APRN, CCNS, CCRN, CNRN
Darcy O'Banion, DNP, APRN, ACCNS-AG
Daphny Peneza, MSN, RN, CNOR, CSSM, FAORN
Ambre Pownall, MSN, RN, APRN, PPCNP-BC
Melinda Sloan, MSN, RN, CNS, ACNP-BC, ANVP-BC, SCRN, CNRN
Andrea Strayer, PhD, AGPCNP-BC, ARNP, CNRN
Deborah Tran, DNP, RN, SCRN, CNRN, NE-BC
Misti Tuppeny, MSN, RN, APRN-CNS, CCRN, CNRN, CCNS
Jennifer Wessol, PhD, RN, CCRN-K, CNRN
Deborah Westover, MSN, RN, CNRN, CNL
Katarzyna Wilk, MSN, APRN-BC, SCRN
Mary Jane Willard, PhD, MBA, MA, RNP, CNRN, CCRN
Elizabeth Winfrey, MSN, RN, CNRN, CCRN, CNL, NPD-BC

Leah Zamora, AANN Staff Liaison

ANA COMMITTEE ON NURSING PRACTICE STANDARDS

Elizabeth O. Dietz, EdD, RN, CS-NP, CSN, FAAN, Co-chair

Mona Pearl Treyball, PhD, RN, CNS, CCRN-K, FAAN, Co-chair

Nena M. Bonuel, PhD, RN, CCRN-E, ACNS-BC, APRN-BC, FNAP

Patricia Bowe, DNP, MS, RN

Ahnyel Burkes, DNP, RN-BC, NEA-BC

Marlissa Esquivel, MSN, RN, AMB-BC

Tonette McAndrew, MPA, BSN, RN

Linda Inez Perkins, MSN, RN-BC

Michael Manasia, MSN, RN, OCN, Alternate

Shelly Wells, PhD, MBA, MS, APRN-CNS, BC-ACNS, ANEF, Alternate

ANA STAFF

James Angelo, MA, Publishing Director

Carol J. Bickford, PhD, NI-BC, CPHIMS, FAMIA, FHIMSS, FAAN, Content editor

Erin E. Walpole, MA, PMP, Production editor

Preface

Neuroscience nursing is a unique and dynamic nursing specialty that addresses the needs and care of individuals with biological, psychological, social, and spiritual alterations because of nervous system conditions (Webb, 2000). Neuroscience nurses are mostly registered nurses (RNs), graduate level prepared nurses, or advanced practice registered nurses (APRNs) but they can also be licensed practical or vocational nurses (LPNs or LVNs). Neuroscience nurses energetically take on the challenges of providing care to neuroscience healthcare consumers, which includes individuals, families, groups, communities, and populations within a complex and constantly changing healthcare environment. The roles of neuroscience RNs and graduate-level prepared RNs, including APRNs, are multifaceted and vibrant. It is crucial for all neuroscience nurses to be aware of the diverse statutes and regulations governing their practice and be able to perform within their defined scopes of practice. This critical foundational document serves to assist neuroscience nurses across any role type in developing their practice.

Setting the Stage

FOUNDATIONAL DOCUMENTS

Neuroscience Nursing: Scope and Standards of Practice describes components of competent nursing practice and professional performance in the specialized field of neuroscience nursing. This document outlines the expectations of the neuroscience nurse professional role, identifies the scope of practice, and presents the standards of professional nursing practice with accompanying competencies for all neuroscience nurses. There are several key foundational resources that inform and guide neuroscience nursing practice in the United States. First, tenets of an ethical framework for neuroscience nurses practicing across all roles, settings, and levels of practice are identified through the *Code of Ethics for Nurses with Interpretive Statements* (American Nurses Association [ANA], 2015). Another significant foundational document is *Nursing's Social Policy Statement: The Essence of the Profession* (ANA, 2010), which conceptualizes nursing practice and describes the social context of nursing. The final foundational resource is *Nursing: Scope and Standards of Practice, Fourth Edition* (ANA, 2021). The scope and standards of neuroscience nursing practice have been developed from these documents.

AUDIENCE

Both RNs and graduate-level prepared RNs, including APRNs, in this exceptional neuroscience nursing specialty constitute the primary audience for this professional resource. Interprofessional colleagues, as well as administrators practicing in healthcare systems, government agencies, and private organizations, will find this a valuable reference in understanding the roles of all neuroscience nurses. In addition, individuals, families, communities, and populations using neuroscience nursing services can use this document to better understand what comprises the practice of neuroscience nursing and who its members are. Finally, legislators, regulators, legal counsel, and the judiciary system may wish to reference this document to better understand what constitutes the practice of neuroscience nursing.

Definitions and Distinguishing Characteristics of Neuroscience Nursing Practice

DEFINITIONS

"*Nursing* integrates the art and science of caring and focuses on the protection, promotion, and optimization of health and human functioning, prevention of illness and injury, and alleviation of suffering through compassionate presence. Nursing is the diagnosis and treatment of human responses, and advocacy in the care of individuals, families, groups, communities, and populations in recognition of the connection of all humanity" (ANA, 2021, p. 1).

Neuroscience nursing is a unique nursing specialty that integrates the art and science of caring while addressing the needs and care of individuals with biological, psychological, social, and spiritual alterations because of nervous system conditions (Webb, 2000). This encompasses all levels of human existence, from basic bodily functions to advanced processes of the human mind. Neuroscience nurses identify and treat human responses to actual or potential health problems related to phenomena affected by nervous system conditions. Phenomena addressed within the context of neuroscience nursing practice include consciousness and cognition, communication, affiliate relationships, mobility, rest and sleep, sensation, elimination, sexuality, self-care, and integrated regulation. In addition, neuroscience nurses teach about preventing neurological injury or illness, conduct research, provide management services, and facilitate quality improvement for individuals with neurological diseases and conditions (Olson, 2017). Recipients of neuroscience nursing care are individuals with potential or actual nervous system conditions, their families and support persons, and the society in which they live.

DISTINGUISHING CHARACTERISTICS

The American Nurses Association (ANA, 2021) identifies essential features of nursing and nursing practice.

Nursing

- Integrates the art and science of caring. In neuroscience nursing, integrating art and science are critical when individuals are unable to speak for themselves due to altered consciousness, cognition, or communication.
- Protects, promotes, and optimizes health and human functioning. In neuroscience nursing, this may include assessment and optimization of environmental adaptations in response to new or prolonged neurological changes.
- Prevents illness and injury. Neuroscience nurses individualize nursing care and education for individuals and caregivers based on assessment of their needs.
- Facilitates healing. Neuroscience nurses are adept at critically distinguishing, analyzing, and communicating the significance of findings from the neurologic exams they conduct.
- Alleviates suffering through compassionate presence. Neuroscience nurses acknowledge and attend with compassion to the unique, multidimensional patient, family, or healthcare clinician needs that arise from experiencing a neurologic illness or injury or caring for someone with a neurological illness or injury.

Nursing is

- The diagnosis and treatment of human responses, and
- Advocacy in the care of individuals, families, groups, communities, and populations in recognition of the connection of all humanity.

Specific phenomena defined by the American Association of Neuroscience Nurses (AANN) that comprise the domains of neuroscience nursing include

- *Consciousness and cognition*: the awareness of and interaction with the surrounding environment, as well as higher thought processes; alterations include problems such as coma, memory impairment, and seizure sequelae;
- *Communication*: the language of interaction with others; alterations include language impairments secondary to aphasias or dysarthria;
- *Affiliate relationships*: the ability to form and maintain social support relationships; alterations include social isolation and role changes secondary to nervous system disease;
- *Mobility*: the ability to move freely within the environment; alterations include various forms of paralysis and paresthesia;
- *Rest and sleep*: phenomena necessary for restorative function; alterations include the spectrum of sleep disorders;
- *Sensation*: the ability to sense and distinguish internal and external stimuli; alterations include decreased sensation and pain;
- *Elimination*: bodily excretion of waste products; alterations include bowel and bladder dysfunction secondary to nervous system disease;
- *Sexuality*: the ability to interact and maintain a sexual relationship; alterations include sexual dysfunction secondary to nervous system disease;

- *Self-care*: the ability to provide for one's basic needs; alterations include the inability to care for oneself; and
- *Integrated regulation*: the interrelationship between the nervous system and other body systems; alterations include loss of regulatory control (Stewart-Amidei & Kunkel, 2000).

HISTORICAL PERSPECTIVE ON NEUROSCIENCE NURSING STANDARDS AND EVOLUTION OF PRACTICE

In the mid-twentieth century and beyond, advances in medical treatment and healthcare technology led to the evolution of nursing specialties. Specialized education, training, and certification ensued in both traditional and novel areas of clinical practice, such as neuroscience nursing. The exciting area of neuroscience nursing was formalized as a specialty in 1968, with the formation of the AANN, then named the American Association of Neurosurgical Nurses. In 1985, the organization's name was changed to the American Association of Neuroscience Nurses to better reflect the diversity of practice of its members.

A statement of the standards of neurologic and neurosurgical nursing practice was first completed in 1977 and approved by the executive committee of the ANA's division of medical-surgical nursing practice and the AANN. A separate statement of neuroscience nursing's scope of practice was first completed in 1986 by the AANN Nursing Practice Committee. This document served to describe the parameters of nursing practice for the specialty, identify the populations served and practice settings, and distinguish qualifications of nurses in the specialty and the type of care rendered to individuals. This description was useful to the neuroscience nurse in defining goals and to the public for clarifying expectations.

In 1993, the standards and scope of practice statements were combined into a single document and updated to address expanded options for neuroscience nursing in the 1990s. In 2002, the third revision, *Scope and Standards of Neuroscience Nursing Practice*, reflected practice evolutions at the beginning of the new millennium. The borders of nursing practice have grown in recent years with potential for continued change with ongoing healthcare reforms. A renewed emphasis is placed on care of individuals across the lifespan and a spectrum of health states rather than focusing on episodes of illness.

Neuroscience nursing practice has evolved along with clinical advances. Previously, neuroscience nursing care focused primarily on symptom management and prevention of secondary complications. While these approaches continue to be necessary, advancements have offered new hope for persons who experience many neurological conditions, incidents, situations, or episodes. For example, in recent decades, care of the patient with multiple sclerosis has evolved from symptomatic care to educating individuals and caregivers about the many pharmacologic agents available. A particular challenge for this population is self-administration of immunomodulating drugs, which neuroscience nurses may help to facilitate.

Another example relates to the advancement of care of the patient who has had a stroke. Neuroscience nurses are now vital members of the interdisciplinary teams that are improving outcomes for individuals with stroke by participating in the delivery of thrombolytic and interventional endovascular therapies. Neuroscience nursing practice also extends to education geared toward early recognition of stroke symptoms. Advances in clinical monitoring, including intracranial pressure monitoring and brain tissue oxygenation monitoring, have allowed neuroscience nurses to become more skilled in applying data about neurologic function to the plan of care.

Neuroscience nursing research findings have contributed to improved outcomes for children with seizures and epilepsy, families of persons with brain tumors, and patients with many other neurological conditions, incidents, situations, or episodes.

As neuroscience nursing evolved as a unique specialty, so have practice opportunities for APRNs. Increased availability of advanced education combined with the shortage of primary and specialty care providers, the need to improve quality of care, restricted residency hours, and promotion of cost-effective care have led to increasing use of APRNs. The number of neuroscience APRNs has grown in recent decades, reflecting the complexity and diversity of the field. *Neuroscience Nursing: Scope and Standards of Practice, Second Edition*, a collaboration between AANN and ANA, was the first to incorporate neuroscience APRNs nursing scope and standards content. In 2009, work began on a stand-alone scope of practice and standards document for APRNs (Stewart-Amidei et al., 2010).

Neuroscience APRNs currently practice across the lifespan and along the continuum of care. While all the innovative areas APRNs practice in are too numerous to include, a few examples are provided. One group reported on providing a pediatric palliative care program for families of children with medical complexities including neurologic and neuromuscular conditions (Pituch et al., 2022). Another group reported on implementing an APRN-led clinic to improve follow-up care for patients who had an ischemic stroke (Mitchell et al., 2022).

As the number and opportunities for acute care nurse practitioners have increased, the successful integration of these types of providers into the healthcare setting has been a challenge. In neurocritical care, APRNs have been instrumental in role development, implementation, and evaluation to optimize the performance of their dynamic roles in intensive care settings. APRNs in neurocritical care have been leaders in expanding and enhancing patient care within the medical practice and collaborating with physicians and other clinicians to provide a full scope of patients care (Yeager, 2009).

Neuroscience Nursing's Scope and Standards of Practice

DESCRIPTION OF THE SCOPE OF NEUROSCIENCE NURSING PRACTICE

The specialty of neuroscience nursing encompasses a broad range of nursing practice. This scope of practice statement describes the who, what, where, when, why, and how associated with neuroscience nursing practice and roles. Neuroscience nurses provide care to individuals at risk for or experiencing problems due to a neurologic condition, their families, and the communities in which they live. Neuroscience nurses provide care across the lifespan. Care during or following neurologic conditions includes, but is not limited to, attention to communication and advance care planning, coordination and transitions of care, and pain and symptom management. Furthermore, neuroscience nurses incorporate three aspects of palliative nursing into their practice: communication and advance care planning, coordination and transitions of care, and pain and symptom management. Major disease categories or conditions that concern neuroscience nurses include degenerative diseases (such as multiple sclerosis and Alzheimer's disease), tumors of the nervous system, neuromuscular diseases (such as myasthenia gravis), traumatic injury to the brain or spine, stroke and other cerebrovascular diseases, seizures/epilepsy, pain, diseases of the spine, movement disorders (such as Parkinson's disease and dystonia), and developmental problems of the nervous system (Hickey & Strayer, 2020). Neuroscience nurses also focus on preventing nervous system conditions through health promotion, community education, and research. The depth and breadth to which individual neuroscience nurses engage in the total scope of neuroscience nursing practice depends on their education, experience, role, work environment, and regulatory bodies. This is addressed in greater detail later in this document.

Neuroscience nursing is built on a core body of knowledge that reflects its dual components of science and art (Hickey & Strayer, 2020). Neuroscience nursing requires judgment and skill based on principles of the biological, physical, psychological, behavioral, and social sciences, with specific focus on neurologic function. Neuroscience nurses employ critical thinking to integrate objective data with knowledge gained from assessing an individuals' subjective experiences. Neuroscience nurses use critical thinking to apply the best available evidence and research data to diagnosis and treatment. Neuroscience nurses continually evaluate quality and effectiveness of nursing practice and seek to optimize outcomes.

The Science of Neuroscience Nursing

Neuroscience nurses, as practice scholars, utilize science and engage in clinical science as a basis of evidence-based practice and care (Hickey et al., 2019). The science of neuroscience nursing is based on an analytical framework of critical thinking composed of assessment, diagnosis, and identification of outcomes, planning, implementation, and evaluation. This is known as the nursing process. These steps serve as the foundation of clinical decision-making and support evidence-based practice. Wherever they practice, neuroscience nurses use the nursing process and other types of critical thinking to respond to the needs of the populations they serve. Neuroscience nurses use strategies that support optimal outcomes most appropriate to the patient or situation, being mindful of resource utilization and conservation.

Neuroscience nurses rely on the application of scientific evidence to guide their policies and practices, but also as a way of quantifying nurses' impact on individual health outcomes. For example, neuroscience nurses have used a bundled approach to improve the recognition and time-to-treatment for strokes that occur in the hospital (Drollinger & Prasun, 2023). An example of neuroscience nurses' leadership in the area of evidence translation and practice implementation is the development of the

AANN Clinical Practice Guidelines series, which provides evidence-based recommendations for the care of individuals with specific conditions, such as traumatic brain injury or brain tumor, or practices such as mobilization of individuals with neurologic injury (AANN, 2012; 2014; 2021). Early mobilization of patients with neurologic conditions in intensive care units has been a recent area of focus, in particular with patients who have external ventricular drains in place or are mechanically ventilated (AANN. 2021; Moyer et al., 2021).

Neuroscience nurses also generate new knowledge in their field through scientific research. AANN has periodically set research priorities, with the aim of advancing the science and practice of neuroscience nursing. Most recently an AANN task force used the Delphi technique to identify impactful neuroscience nursing research categories and topics (Bautista et al., 2022). The following were selected by neuroscience nurse experts:

- *Assessment*: Assessment parameters for specific neurological conditions
- *Biomarkers*
  - Recovery from various relevant neurologic injury/disease processes
  - Intervention efficacy in various relevant neurologic injury/disease
  - Neuro/oncology and targeted treatments
- *Nursing Care Outcomes*
  - Interventions to improve outcomes
  - Care across a spectrum of neuroscience problems
  - ICP Monitoring
  - Neuro Infections
  - Degenerative Spine Disease
  - Parkinson's Disease
  - Care across the lifespan
  - Pediatric patients
  - *Quality of Life*: Relevant neurologic injury/disease populations
  - *Technology*: Symptom monitoring

The following strategies have been identified to improve the overall impact of neuroscience nursing research in all topic areas (Bautista et al., 2022):

- Evaluate specific neuroscience nursing interventions using rigorous scientific designs
- Address the lifespan and continuum of patient populations cared for by neuroscience nurses
- Define neuroscience nursing sensitive outcomes in order to test the effectiveness of interventions as compared to describing current state
- Incorporate biomarkers as a measure of response to nursing and medical interventions
- Expand neuroscience nursing in areas of emerging trends (e.g., caregivers, technology, biomarkers)

The Art of Neuroscience Nursing

The art of neuroscience nursing is based on compassion and respect for human dignity. A compassionate approach to patient care mandates that care is provided competently, provided and accomplished through both independent practice and partnerships. Collaboration may occur between professional colleagues or with healthcare consumers. The art of caring is central to neuroscience nursing practice and is represented in the personal relationship between the nurse and the patient. The art of caring goes beyond emotional human connections, extending to the ability to respond to the human aspects of health and illness during critical moments in a way that promotes healing and social justice.

The art of neuroscience nursing embraces dynamic processes that affect the human person, including, for example, spirituality, healing, empathy, mutual respect, and compassion. These intangible aspects are fostered by compassion, helping, listening, mentoring, coaching, teaching, exploring, being present, supporting, touching, intuition, empathy, service, cultural competence, tolerance, acceptance, nurturing, mutually creating, and conflict resolution.

Neuroscience nursing focuses on the promotion and maintenance of health and the prevention or resolution of disease, illness, or disability. Human needs are met in the context of a culturally sensitive, caring, and personal relationship by the neuroscience nurse. Neuroscience nursing includes the diagnosis and treatment of human responses to actual or potential health problems. Neuroscience nurses employ practices that are restorative, supportive, and promotive in nature:

- *Restorative* practices modify the impact of neurologic illness or disease.
- *Supportive* practices are oriented toward modification of relationships or the environment to support health.
- *Promotive* practices mobilize healthy patterns of living, foster personal and family development, and support self-defined goals of individuals, families, communities, and populations.

DEVELOPMENT AND FUNCTION OF NURSING STANDARDS

The standards of neuroscience nursing practice are authoritative statements of the duties that all neuroscience nurses, regardless of role or population, are expected to competently perform (ANA, 2021). The standards published herein may be utilized as evidence of a legal standard of care. The standards are subject to change with the dynamics of the neuroscience nursing specialty—as new patterns of professional practice are developed and accepted by neuroscience nurses, the education community, and the public—and as changes in societal trends occur.

This document includes 18 standard statements that provide the neuroscience nurse with a framework for outlining an expansive scope of practice. The language is intentionally broad and serves to paint an overall picture of practice. The roles and activities of the neuroscience nurse may be specific to practice setting and directed by state, institution, or group practice requirements. The standard statements enclosed in this document perform optimally when tailored and applied to the specifics of a particular nursing practice focus or setting.

Each standard statement is accompanied by several basic competencies. The competency statements, in turn, may be further specified according to practice setting. Competencies are specific, measurable elements that interpret, explain, and facilitate practical use of a standard. The competencies may be used to demonstrate evidence of compliance with individual standards but are not exhaustive and may be circumstantial. For example, the plan of care (Standard 4. Planning) may not be able to be developed with or communicated to the unresponsive patient who has no identified family caregiver.

Competencies may be used by neuroscience nurses to appraise professional performance and identify content for academic and continuing education curricula. Neuroscience nurses can also use the competencies to inform others of practice expectations.

THE NURSING PROCESS

Neuroscience nurses use the nursing process to deliver care. The nursing process is often conceptualized linearly, moving from assessment to diagnosis, outcomes identification, planning, implementation, and evaluation. However, these steps are often necessarily interrelated, as one step may inform another (Figure 1; ANA, 2015).

The Neuroscience Nursing Standards of Practice coincide with the steps of the nursing process. The nursing process begins with assessment. These standards focus specifically on neurologic assessment. Data gathered from the neurologic assessment are used to plan and implement nursing interventions specific to the patient's neurologic condition. Interventions may support bodily functions and promote healing and recovery of the acutely ill, enhance adaptation to persistent neurologic deficits for the chronically ill, facilitate patient and family coping, and teach individuals and their families about disease processes, adaptation techniques, and therapies. The neuroscience nurse evaluates patient outcomes on an ongoing basis and revises the care plan as necessary. Further, application of clinically relevant research findings promotes evidence-based care and development of creative, therapeutic nursing interventions to improve outcomes for individuals with neurologic conditions.

Ethical principles are applied in any care rendered. Similarly, the Neuroscience Nursing Standards of Professional Performance relate to how the professional nurse adheres to the Neuroscience Nursing Standards of Practice, completes the nursing process, and addresses other practice issues and concerns (ANA, 2021).

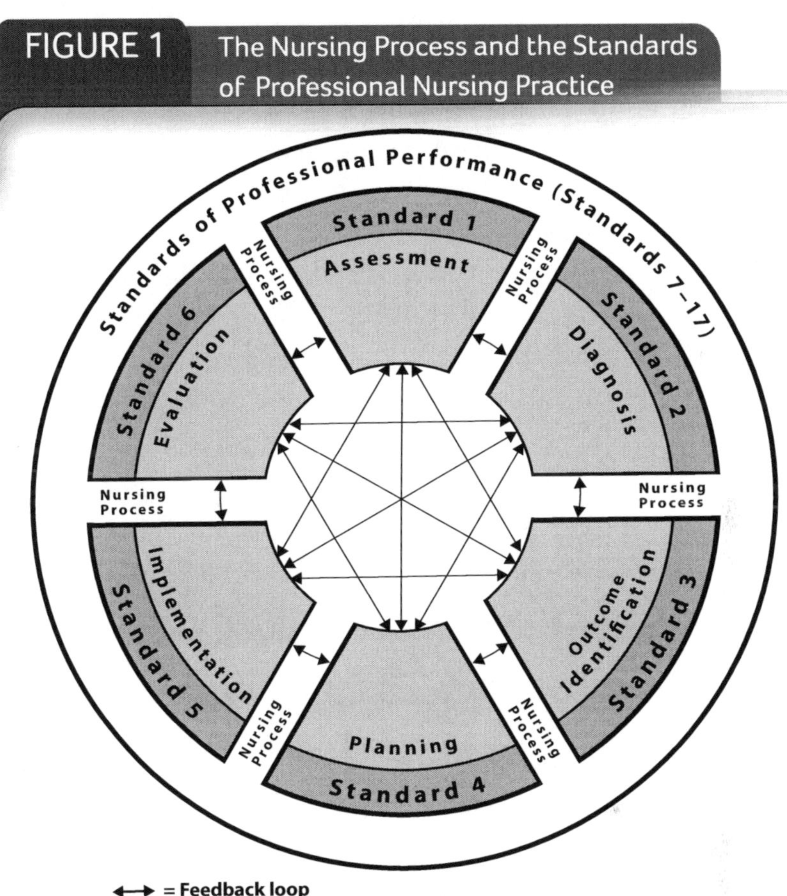

◄──► = Feedback loop

From: *Nursing Scope and Standards of Practice* (3rd ed., p. 14), American Nurses Association, 2015.

TENETS OF NEUROSCIENCE NURSING PRACTICE

Four tenets characterize contemporary neuroscience nursing practice, and are reflective of nursing practice as a whole:

1. Neuroscience Nursing Practice Is Individualized

Neuroscience nursing practice respects diversity and is individualized to meet the unique needs of the patient. The patient is defined as the individual with or at risk for a neurologic condition, and their family, group, community, or population who is the focus of attention and to whom the neuroscience nurse is providing services as sanctioned by state regulatory bodies. For example, the neuroscience nurse recognizes that each person with a brain tumor or stroke will present different signs and symptoms, and care must be individualized according to identified needs.

Furthermore, neuroscience nurses use theoretical and evidence-based knowledge to advocate for and collaborate with individuals in assessing, diagnosing, and identifying outcomes, and planning, implementing, and evaluating individualized care. Nursing interventions are intended to incorporate a shared decision-making model that prioritizes individualized care and contributes to quality outcomes. Critical thinking underlies each step of the nursing, problem-solving, and decision-making processes. The nursing process is cyclical and dynamic, with each step informing both the previous step and the succeeding step. The nursing process is also patient centered, interpersonal, collaborative, and universally applicable.

2. Neuroscience Nurses Coordinate Care by Establishing Partnerships

Neuroscience nurses establish partnerships with persons, families, communities, support systems, and other providers, utilizing in-person and electronic communication methods to reach a shared goal of delivering healthcare. Collaborative, interprofessional team planning is based on recognition of each discipline's value and contributions, mutual trust, respect, open discussion, and shared decision-making. Neuroscience nurses frequently partner with other disciplines, such as physical therapy, occupational therapy, and speech therapy, to optimize care. One example is the use of an interprofessional approach to provide optimal care for a vulnerable veteran population with amyotrophic lateral sclerosis (Jaffa et al., 2017). Care may also be coordinated with other specialties, including (but not limited to) pediatrics, psychiatry, or geriatrics. Neuroscience nurses may need to collaborate with any specialty regarding a neuroscience patient and maintain knowledge in emerging specialties to optimize patient care.

3. Caring and Health Are Central to the Practice of Neuroscience Nursing

Professional nursing promotes healing and health in a way that builds a relationship between the neuroscience nurse and individuals. "Caring is a conscious judgment that manifests itself in concrete acts, interpersonally, verbally, and non-verbally" (Gallagher-Lepak & Kubsch, 2009, p. 171). Neuroscience nurses communicate caring through touch, verbal communication, and nonverbal behaviors while also promoting self-care, environmental care, and societal care.

4. A Strong Link Exists Between the Professional Work Environment and Neuroscience Nurses' Ability to Provide Quality Patient Care and Achieve Optimal Patient Outcomes

Neuroscience nurses have an ethical obligation to maintain and improve healthcare environments that are conducive to providing quality healthcare (ANA, 2010). Elements of a healthy work environment have been extensively studied and document the relationship between effective practice and quality of the work environment. Neuroscience nurses must maintain and improve the healthcare environment for both nurses and individuals in order to prevent injury and illness as well as promote health.

HEALTHY WORK ENVIRONMENTS FOR NEUROSCIENCE NURSES

Negative, demoralizing, and unsafe conditions in the workplace, emanating from a physical or psychologically unhealthy environment, contribute to nursing errors, ineffective delivery of care, conflict, and stress among healthcare teams and those they serve. The neuroscience nurse is expected to contribute toward the reduction or elimination of physical and psychological health risks in the employment setting, thus creating a healthy work environment.

The Institute of Medicine (IOM) reported that safety and quality problems exist when dedicated health professionals work within systems that neither prepare nor support them in achieving optimal patient care outcomes (2004). Rapid changes, such as reimbursement modification and cost-containment efforts, new healthcare technologies, and changes in the healthcare workforce, have influenced the work and work environment for all nurses. Concentrating on key aspects of the work environment, encompassing people, physical places, and tools, can enhance healthcare working conditions and improve safety. Key aspects include utilizing transformational leadership and evidence-based care management, maximizing workforce capability, creating and sustaining a culture of safety and research, evaluating workspace design and redesign to prevent and mitigate errors, addressing potential pollutants in the work environment, and promoting the effective use of telecommunications.

Creating and maintaining a healthy work environment requires effort. Establishing and maintaining a healthy work environment requires all nurses, not only neuroscience nurses, to

- Be proficient in skilled communication;
- Foster true collaboration with partners across all disciplines;
- Be effective decision-makers in policy, in directing and evaluating clinical care, and in leading organizations;
- Ensure appropriate staffing that matches nurse competencies to patient needs;
- Foster meaningful recognition of the value of self and others; and
- Embrace the role of a leader in creating and sustaining a healthy work environment.

The Magnet Recognition Program (ANCC, 2014; 2023) also addresses the professional work environment, requiring that Magnet-designated facilities adhere to the model components of transformational leadership, structured empowerment, exemplary professional practice, new knowledge, innovation and improvements, and empirical quality results.

These collective principles of a healthy employment environment apply to neuroscience nurses who work in any healthcare environment. This requires the neuroscience nurse to collaborate often and well, to communicate the important contributions of nursing to the health and well-being of those with neurologic conditions, and to assume leadership roles in settings where they are employed.

Issues specific to a healthy work environment for neuroscience nurses relate to the nature of the intense issues and phenomena encountered in neuroscience practice. While many challenges exist in all areas of nursing practice, neuroscience nurses may more frequently encounter issues that affect their emotional health. One research study reported that the implementation of resilience rooms (dedicated spaces for nurses to decompress) in neuroscience units helped to decrease emotional distress and burnout in a sample of 396 neuroscience nurses (Prendergast et al., 2023). Thus, neuroscience nurses continue to strive toward creating healthy work environments.

APPLICATION OF PROVISIONS OF THE *CODE OF ETHICS FOR NURSES*

Neuroscience nurses incorporate the nine provisions of the *Code of Ethics for Nurses* (ANA, 2015). The following are examples of how the neuroscience professional incorporates these provisions:

> Provision 1: The neuroscience nurse practices with compassion and respect for the inherent dignity, worth, and unique attributes of every person.

The neuroscience nurse focuses on helping individuals meet their needs, including physical, emotional, cognitive, social, and spiritual needs. Each patient is an individual, and care must be tailored to meet the healthcare needs encompassing all aspects of an individual's life, culture, and community.

> Provision 2: The neuroscience nurse's primary commitment is to the patient, whether an individual, family, group, community, or population.

The neuroscience nurse always maintains professional boundaries with their patients, whether individuals, families, groups, communities, or a population. The neuroscience nurse is always alert for potential conflicts of interest that may affect individuals and disclose inappropriate information. The neuroscience nurse always prioritizes the well-being of their patient, whether an individual, family, group, community, or population.

The neuroscience nurse cares for the patient without judgment. In addition, the neuroscience nurse provides holistic and altruistic care to bring the patient to utmost health and improve their quality of life. Neuroscience nurses provide creative critical thinking for positive and safe outcomes. The neuroscience nurse demonstrates positive demeanor while developing trust and mutual respect, and while incorporating healing interactions that benefit the patient.

The neuroscience nurse recognizes their role in the nursing profession and their responsibility to provide competent care to individuals with neurological conditions, guided by the laws of their state and protocols of their facility. The neuroscience nurse takes actions such as advocating at the patient level, as well as using their expertise in the profession to provide guidance for practice changes.

The neuroscience nurse maintains personal health, safety, and overall physical, emotional, psychological, and spiritual well-being to mitigate burnout and fatigue. The neuroscience nurse maintains personal and professional integrity and wholeness of character to avoid endangering a patient, family, community, or nursing practice. The neuroscience nurse engages in activities to increase their knowledge and maintain competence to promote personal and professional growth to reciprocate and interact in the world in which they live.

The neuroscience nurse engages in skilled communication and fosters collaboration with multiple disciplines to promote autonomy within the healthcare environment. The neuroscience nurse, individually and as part of a team, demonstrates integrity and respect in the practice of nursing, in which solutions and concerns are addressed to promote self-worth and respect.

Persons with a neurologic condition are often unable to move independently and may require a great deal of physical assistance, thereby placing the neuroscience nurse at risk for injury. Neuroscience nurses can use special equipment, including mechanical lifts, or services such as lift teams to protect themselves. Persons with neurologic conditions may present unfavorable behaviors that can injure themselves, family members, or healthcare staff. Within their work environment, neuroscience nurses promote safety by observing for escalating violent behaviors, working as a team to diffuse violent behaviors, and educating family members and coworkers about how to best deal with safety concerns.

In 2017, to advance the profession of neuroscience nursing, the AANN created a standing committee on clinical science. The objective of the committee is to advance clinical science through research, scholarly inquiry, and quality. Key achievements of this committee have been to define clinical science (Hickey et al., 2019) and the set research priorities for neuroscience nursing (Bautista et al., 2022).

Based on evidence, the neuroscience nurse provides care for all individuals regardless of race, color, sex, national origin, age, disability, genetic information, creed, or socioeconomic status, with consideration of cultural values that can promote or hinder health and wellness. The neuroscience nurse advocates on behalf of all individuals for best practice, care access (inclusive of preventive, episodic, and chronic care), healthy living environments, and health education.

> Provision 9: The profession of nursing, collectively through its professional organizations, must articulate nursing values, maintain the integrity of the profession, and integrate principles of social justice into nursing and health policy.

The neuroscience nurse works collectively through their professional association, AANN (a premier organizational affiliate of the ANA), to articulate neuroscience nursing values, maintain the integrity of the profession, and integrate principles of social justice into nursing and health policy.

SCHOLARSHIP IN NEUROSCIENCE NURSING

Scholarship is a hallmark of all professions and includes research and practice scholarship. Building the science for practice and care is a major responsibility of each profession. AANN has assumed this responsibility in numerous ways: publishing clinical practice guidelines and articles to inform the readership about knowledge development and its application to practice, supporting the application of neuroscience nursing knowledge through active engagement with other professional organizations focused on neuroscience patient care, and influencing health policy to address the needs of neuroscience patients and practice. It is through these efforts that the scholarship of neuroscience nursing is framed. AANN works synergistically with the American Board of Neuroscience Nursing (ABNN) and the Agnes Marshall Walker Foundation (AMWF) through a shared vision that together AANN, ABNN, and AMWF are the three pillars driving neuroscience nursing excellence and scholarship (Hickey et al., 2019).

MODEL OF PROFESSIONAL PRACTICE REGULATION

The Model Representing Regulation of Professional Nursing Practice (Figure 2) reaffirms the profession's focus on the safety, quality, and evidence-base of nursing practice. The *Neuroscience Nursing: Scope and Standards of Practice* are derived from this model.

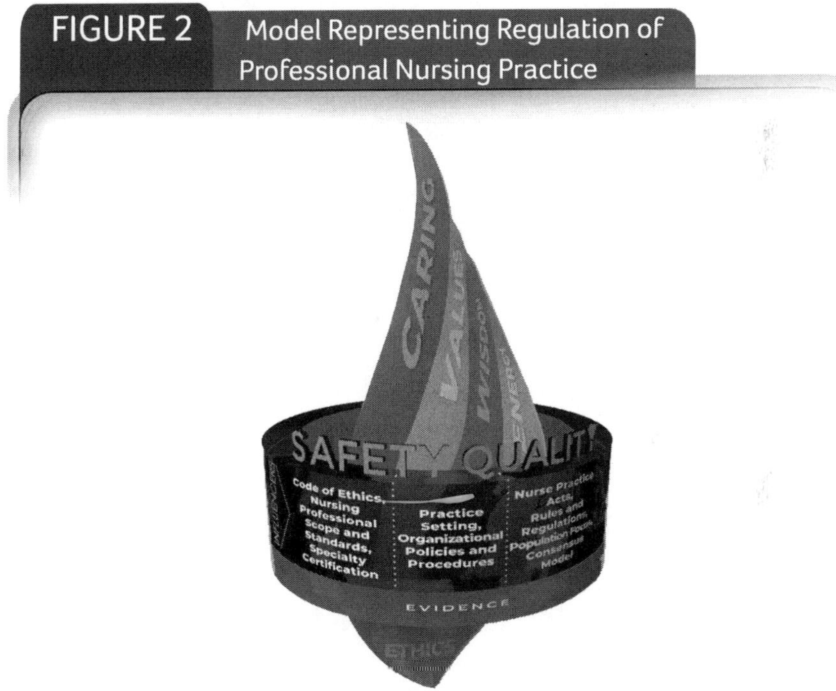

FIGURE 2 Model Representing Regulation of Professional Nursing Practice

From American Nurses Association, 2021.

Overview of the Standards of Neuroscience Nursing Practice

The Standards of Neuroscience Nursing Practice are composed of the Standards of Practice and the Standards of Professional Performance.

PROFESSIONAL COMPETENCE IN NEUROSCIENCE NURSING PRACTICE

The public has a right to expect neuroscience nurses to demonstrate professional competence throughout their careers. Neuroscience nurses are individually responsible and accountable for maintaining professional competence. It is the nurse's professional responsibility to shape and guide the process that assures neuroscience nurse competence. Regulatory agencies define minimal standards of competence to protect the public. The employer is responsible and accountable to provide a practice environment conducive to competent practice. Assurance of competence is the shared responsibility of the profession, individual nurses, professional organizations, credentialing and certification entities, regulatory agencies, employers, and other key stakeholders (AANN, 2015; ANA, 2014).

AANN believes that, in the practice of neuroscience nursing, competence can be defined, measured, and evaluated. No single evaluation method or tool can guarantee competence (ANA, 2014, p. 6). Competence is situational and dynamic; it is both an outcome and an ongoing process. Context determines what competencies are necessary.

Definitions and Concepts Related to Neuroscience Nursing Competence

Several terms and ideas are central to the discussion of competence:

- An individual who demonstrates competence is performing at an expected level
- A *competency* is an expected level of performance that integrates knowledge, skills, abilities, and judgment
- Integration of knowledge, skills, abilities, and judgment occurs in formal, informal, and reflective learning experiences
- Knowledge encompasses thinking, understanding of science and humanities, professional standards of practice, and insights gained from context, practical experiences, personal capabilities, and leadership performance
- Skills include psychomotor, communication, interpersonal, and diagnostic skills
- Ability is the capacity to act effectively. It requires listening, integrity, knowledge of one's strengths and weaknesses, positive self-regard, emotional intelligence, and openness to feedback
- Judgment includes critical thinking, problem solving, ethical reasoning, and decision-making (ANA, 2014)

Competence and Competency in Neuroscience Nursing Practice

Competent neuroscience nursing practice can be influenced by the nature of the situation, which includes consideration of the setting, resources, and person. Situations can either enhance or detract from the neuroscience nurse's ability to perform. All neuroscience nurses influence factors that facilitate and enhance competent practice. Similarly, neuroscience nurses seek to address barriers that constrain competent practice. The expected level of performance reflects variability depending upon context and the selected competency framework or model.

The ability to perform at the expected level requires a process of lifelong learning. All neuroscience nurses must continually reassess their competencies and identify needs for additional knowledge, skills, personal growth, and integrative learning experiences.

Evaluating Competence

Competence in neuroscience nursing practice must be evaluated by the individual nurse (self-assessment), nurse peers, and nurses in the roles of supervisor, coach, mentor, clinical educator, or preceptor. In addition, other aspects of neuroscience nursing performance may be evaluated by professional colleagues and healthcare consumers.

Competence can be evaluated by using tools that capture objective and subjective data about the individual's knowledge base and actual performance and that are appropriate for the specific situation and the desired outcome of the competence evaluation. "However, no single evaluation tool or method can guarantee competence" (ANA, 2014, p. 6).

PROFESSIONAL NEUROSCIENCE NURSES TODAY

Statistical Snapshot

Neuroscience nurses may choose membership in the organization supporting their specialty, AANN. Statistics on neuroscience nurses are based on AANN membership and certification rates, although it is important to acknowledge that not all neuroscience nurses are members of the organization. AANN membership is composed of nearly 5,000 RNs and APRNs. AANN members primarily work in academic medical centers, but often work in community hospitals, ambulatory or rehabilitation settings, or in private practices. Primary practice areas for neuroscience nurses are medical-surgical and critical care units, although some work in outpatient and perioperative areas.

Neuroscience nurses work with healthcare consumers and their families across the lifespan as neurologic conditions may occur at any age. Neuroscience nurses in specialty practice represent the full spectrum from novice to expert. AANN membership is not prerequisite to neuroscience nursing certification. There are nearly 4,000 RNs with the Certified Neuroscience Registered Nurse (CNRN) credential and more than 6,600 RNs with the Stroke Certified Registered Nurse (SCRN) credential.

Continuing the profession depends on nursing education, appropriate organization of nursing services, continued expansion of nursing knowledge, and policy development and adoption. Such initiatives demand that neuroscience nurses be adequately prepared for specialty practice. As specialists in their profession, neuroscience nurses collaborate, consult, and serve as liaisons, bridging the role of the neuroscience nurse with that of other professions and specialties. For example, neuroscience nurses closely align with and interact with neurovascular nurses to provide high quality, evidence-based nursing care (ANA, 2023). As collaborators and specialists, neuroscience nurses help to delineate nursing's professional role in society.

Licensure and Education of Neuroscience Nurses

The neuroscience nurse is licensed as a registered nurse and authorized to practice nursing by a state, commonwealth, or territory. Professional healthcare licensure is established by each jurisdiction to protect public safety and authorizes professional practice. For this reason, the requirements for RN and APRN licensure vary widely.

The neuroscience RN is educationally prepared for competent practice at the novice level upon graduation from an accredited school or college of nursing and qualified by national examination for RN licensure. AANN affirms the baccalaureate degree in nursing (BSN) as the preferred educational preparation for entry into nursing practice (Hinkle et al., 2012; Madden et al., 2017). Neuroscience nurses who have not acquired a BSN are encouraged to meet these qualifications.

Through orientation, continuing education, guided practice, and mentorship, nurses develop the specialized body of knowledge and experience that characterizes neuroscience nursing practice. Credentialing is one way to acknowledge such specialized knowledge and experience.

Credentialing organizations may mandate specific nursing educational requirements, as well as timely demonstration of knowledge and experience in specialty practice. RNs who work in neuroscience nursing may choose to test their proficiency in neuroscience nursing to become certified. Earned and maintained by nearly 4,000 nurses, the CNRN credential represents specialized experience and knowledge in the care of individuals with neurological trauma and illness. Earned and maintained by more than 6,600 nurses, the SCRN credential formally recognizes the attainment and demonstration of a unique body of knowledge necessary for the practice of stroke nursing. Ongoing certification may be retained for the CNRN and the SCRN either through continuing education or retesting. Appropriate documentation must be maintained. The neuroscience RN may also seek and maintain other professional certifications (AANN, 2015).

New models for educational preparation are constantly evolving in response to the changing healthcare, education, and regulatory practice environments. All neuroscience RNs have the professional responsibility to maintain their competence in practice through ongoing skill development and lifelong learning. AANN offers continuing education through professional conferences and through its journal, *Journal of Neuroscience Nursing*. In some states, continuing education is tied to re-licensure.

Neuroscience Advanced Practice Registered Nurses

The need to ensure patient safety and access to APRNs by aligning education, accreditation, licensure, and certification is delineated by the APRN Joint Dialogue Group (JDG) in the *Consensus Model for APRN Regulation: Licensure, Accreditation, Certification, and Education*. The APRN JDG (2008) defines the APRN as having

- Completed an accredited graduate-level education program with preparation in one of the four recognized APRN roles;
- Passed a national certification examination that measures APRN competencies;
- Acquired advanced clinical knowledge and skills preparing them to provide direct care to healthcare consumers, as well as a component of indirect care;
- A practice that builds on the competencies of the registered nurse;
- Educational preparation to assume responsibility and accountability for health promotion and maintenance as well as the assessment, diagnosis, and management of healthcare consumer problems, including the use and prescription of pharmacologic and non-pharmacologic interventions;
- Clinical experience of sufficient depth and breadth to reflect the intended license;

- Obtained a license to practice as an APRN in one of the four APRN roles: certified registered nurse anesthetist (CRNA), certified nurse-midwife (CNM), clinical nurse specialist (CNS), or nurse practitioner (NP).

The AANN supports the four requirements necessary for regulation of the advanced practice role: licensure, accreditation, certification, and education (APRN JDG, 2008). Advanced Practice Registered Nurse is a regulatory title and, in neuroscience nursing, includes the roles of certified registered nurse anesthetist (CRNA), clinical nurse specialist (CNS), or nurse practitioner (NP). State laws and regulations further define criteria for licensure for the designated scopes of practice.

The neuroscience APRN has a specialized body of knowledge and expanded clinical skills acquired at the graduate level, with the master's degree as the minimum requirement for entry into advanced practice (AACN, 1998). Advanced practice certification via examination through the appropriate nationally recognized organization is a requirement for licensure in most states. The American Nurses Credentialing Center offers multiple certification examinations for NPs and CNSs in addition to other advanced practice examinations (APRN JDG, 2008). The American Academy of Nurse Practitioners offers a variety of certification examinations for nurse practitioners. Specialty nursing certification exams for advanced practice, such as those offered through the Oncology Nursing Certification Corporation, the Pediatric Nursing Credentialing Board and the American Association of Critical Care Nurses Certification Corporation, may also be acceptable for licensure.

ROLES AND RESPONSIBILITIES OF NEUROSCIENCE REGISTERED NURSES

Neuroscience nursing responsibilities focus on the unique problems of healthcare consumers with neurologic conditions, and the primary role is direct care delivery. Beyond direct delivery of care, the neuroscience nurse may assume a variety of roles, such as educator, administrator, researcher, consultant, advocate, and clinical expert. Each role is based upon specific clinical expertise and education. Basic nursing role titles may include staff nurses with varying degrees of advancement.

Neuroscience nurse responsibilities focus on the healthcare consumer with neurologic conditions and include

- Providing age-appropriate as well as culturally- and linguistically-appropriate care;
- Maintaining a safe environment;
- Educating healthcare consumers and their families about health promotion, disease prevention, and treatment modalities;
- Assuring continuity of care;
- Coordinating care across settings and among caregivers;
- Managing information;
- Communicating effectively; and
- Engaging in community outreach to healthcare consumers with neurologic conditions.

Additional responsibilities may be specified by the setting where the neuroscience nurse is employed.

Professionalism is demonstrated by assuming accountability for maintaining excellence in practice through self-motivated ventures and collaborative efforts with other nursing colleagues, organizations, and interprofessional associates. Participation in the specialty's certification process further identifies the nurse's commitment to excellence in neuroscience nursing practice (AANN, 2015).

ROLES AND RESPONSIBILITIES OF NEUROSCIENCE ADVANCED PRACTICE REGISTERED NURSES

Expert clinical practice is the hallmark of advanced practice nursing. Clinical practice involves assessment, diagnosis, and management of patient problems, as well as health promotion. The following are primary generic APRN responsibilities, regardless of specialty (APRN JDG, 2008):

- Plans and coordinates interventions from an interprofessional perspective
- Functions across the healthcare system and works with diverse populations
- Initiates and facilitates quality improvement initiatives
- Facilitates, conducts and promotes utilization of research activities in practice
- Develops education strategies and evaluates effectiveness of educational interventions
- Recommends and influences social and healthcare policies
- Provides consultation to improve care
- Applies legal and ethical standards to complex situations

Each of these responsibilities may be directly applied into specialty practice by the neuroscience APRN (Villanueva et al., 2008). Interventions may occur from an independent or collaborative decision-making position. Specific neuroscience APRN activities may be influenced by workforce fluctuations, development of related healthcare specialties, geographic and economic disparities, economic incentives, and consumer demand. There are many diverse statutes (state, federal, and community) and institutional guidelines which govern APRNs. For those APRNs who are required to practice within a contractual agreement, protocols may be collaboratively developed that address specific responsibilities and expectations (Yeager et al., 2006). Neuroscience APRNs strive to practice to their full potential based on each state's licensure requirements.

NEUROSCIENCE NURSE PRACTICE SETTINGS

Neuroscience nurses practice in a wide range of settings to care for healthcare consumers with nervous system conditions, along with their families or support persons. Multiple practice sites provide care for neuroscience healthcare consumers, including hospitals, outpatient settings, private practice, academic institutions, research facilities, rehabilitation centers, and community settings. Care provision may occur with virtual or telehealth components. Care may have a specific disease focus, such as neuro-oncology; a specialty focus, such as neurosurgery; or a problem focus, such as chronic pain management. Care may be provided across the lifespan, or within a specific age group (children or older adults).

Board certified nurse practitioners or clinical nurse specialists may practice as neuroscience APRNs. The following are examples of advanced practice applications but are by no means exhaustive. The neuroscience APRN may practice in the neurosurgery intensive care unit (ICU), providing direct patient care while mentoring staff nurses and orienting new graduates. Another neuroscience APRN may practice within the pediatric neurosurgery specialty, performing preoperative and postoperative assessments of children or providing direct and indirect care to children with complex neurosurgical needs (e.g., traumatic brain injury, craniotomy for tumor resection, cranial vault remodeling, and neonates with myelomeningocele) in the ICU. A third neuroscience APRN may practice in the clinic setting, providing specialized care to older adults with movement disorders such as Parkinson's disease or myasthenia gravis, managing care for both inpatients and outpatients, or providing stroke screening and implementing stroke prevention initiatives. The neuroscience APRN may also design and implement quality improvement projects to improve population-based outcomes or system processes. Finally, the neuroscience APRN working in the perioperative area may conduct assessments, write orders, and assist the neurosurgical team.

In all the identified settings, practice levels, and roles, the primary intent is to care for, support, teach, and serve as an advocate for the healthcare consumer with a neurologic condition. The goal of all interventions in neuroscience nursing practice is consistent with and flows from that of the entire nursing profession: to provide the highest quality of care to healthcare consumers and achieve a state of wellness consistent with the quality of life desired by the healthcare consumer, which may include a peaceful and dignified death.

NEUROSCIENCE NURSING'S SOCIETAL AND ETHICAL DIMENSIONS

Neuroscience nursing responds to the changing needs of society and the expanding knowledge base of its theoretical and scientific domains. One of neuroscience nursing's objectives is to optimize patient outcomes that maximize quality of life across the entire life span. Neuroscience nurses facilitate the interprofessional and comprehensive care provided by healthcare professionals, paraprofessionals, and volunteers. In other instances, neuroscience nurses engage in consultation with other colleagues to inform decision-making and planning to meet healthcare consumer needs. Neuroscience nurses often participate in interprofessional teams in which overlapping skills complement each member's individual efforts.

All nursing practice, regardless of specialty, role, or setting, is a fundamentally independent practice. Neuroscience nurses are accountable for individual nursing judgments and actions taken during their nursing practice. Therefore, all neuroscience nurses are responsible for assessing individual competence and are committed to the process of lifelong learning. All neuroscience nurses develop and maintain current knowledge and skills through formal and continuing education and by seeking certification.

Neuroscience nurses are bound by the same professional code of ethics (ANA, 2015) that guides all nurses. Neuroscience nurses regulate themselves as individuals through a collegial process of peer review. Peer evaluation fosters the refinement of knowledge, skills, and clinical decision-making at all levels and in all areas of clinical practice. Self-regulation assures performance quality, which is the heart of nursing's social contract (ANA, 2010).

Neuroscience nurses and their professional colleagues exchange knowledge and ideas about how to deliver high-quality healthcare, resulting in constantly changing professional practice boundaries. True collaboration involves recognizing the expertise of others within and outside one's profession and consulting and referring to specialized providers when appropriate. Collaboration also involves some shared functions and a common focus on one overall mission. By necessity, neuroscience nursing's scope of practice has flexible boundaries.

Neuroscience nurses regularly evaluate safety, effectiveness, and cost when planning and delivering nursing care. Nurses recognize that resources are limited and unequally distributed, and that the potential for better access to care requires innovative approaches, such as treating individuals remotely through technology applications. An example of this is the use of telestroke nurses partnering with neuroradiologists to help extend the window of treatment opportunity for patients who have had a stroke (Helms et al., 2023). As members of a profession, neuroscience nurses work toward equitable distribution and availability of healthcare services throughout the nation and the world.

Ethical dimensions of neuroscience nursing practice are influenced by the nature of the phenomena outlining the framework of neuroscience nursing. Individuals cared for by neuroscience nurses may have altered cognition or language impairments that render them vulnerable and unable to vocalize their needs. Neuroscience nurses may serve as patient advocates and play a vital role in facilitating surrogate decision-making on the patient's behalf. Encouraging individuals to formulate advance directives allows individuals to communicate their wishes when they are unable to do so. The potential for irreversible brain injury or progressive neurological deterioration in the population that neuroscience nurses serve poses additional ethical concerns. Neuroscience nurses anticipate these problems and actively participate in discussions about withholding or withdrawal of care by preparing individuals and families to address these issues. For example, when working with a patient with amyotrophic lateral sclerosis, the neuroscience nurse may participate in a discussion with the patient and family about the option of withholding intubation for respiratory distress or explain the life support withdrawl process to the family of a patient who has met the criteria for brain death. Because individuals with neurologic conditions may be left with persistent deficits, neuroscience nurses also play an integral role in determining the need for rehabilitation and assuring access to restorative care.

CONTINUED COMMITMENT TO THE PROFESSION

A continued commitment to the nursing profession requires neuroscience nurses to remain involved in continuous learning and strengthening individual practice within varied practice settings. This may include civic activities, membership in and support of professional associations (such as the AANN), collective bargaining, and workplace advocacy.

Neuroscience nurses promote the health of the individual and society regardless of cultural background, value system, religious belief, gender, sexuality, or disability. Advocacy can also extend beyond the healthcare system to the community and legislative realms in an attempt to create environments that lower health risk and promote equitable health outcomes. Neuroscience nurses commit to their profession by utilizing their skills, knowledge, and abilities to act as visionaries, promoting safe practice environments and supporting resourceful, accessible, and cost-effective delivery of healthcare to serve the ever-changing needs of the population. Ever-evolving technological advances, like artificial intelligence and machine learning, offer neuroscience nurses opportunities to devise new workflows, analytics, and virtual roles in order to enhance patient care. Through traditional and innovative techniques, neuroscience nurses will remain committed to advancing their specialty through quality improvement, nursing research, and implementation of evidence-based practice.

PROFESSIONAL TRENDS AND ISSUES

Neuroscience nursing is evolving and will continue to do so, in conjunction with technological advances, greater scientific understanding, and a rapidly growing research base. Nursing has moved from an era of needing only to provide good, safe, physical care to the patient with severe neurologic conditions to the era of direct translation of research into care. An example of this is the prompt treatment of stroke. Twenty years ago, stroke care consisted of supportive and rehabilitative care only. It is now possible to reverse stroke deficits with early intervention, and neuroscience nurses at all levels of practice play a key role in operationalizing this process.

Another technological advance that neuroscience nurses are integrally involved in is the care of patients with Parkinson's disease and other movement disorders who have had deep brain stimulators surgically implanted. This technology requires much education, monitoring of equipment, and support for patients and their families.

Neuroscience nurses are increasingly involved in research activities, not just as research consumers, but as independent or collaborative researchers. Advances in various branches of science, such as neurogenetics, are rapidly changing the face of neuroscience nursing practice. Genetics may broaden treatment options, and nurses must be aware, not only of the clinical implications, but the ethical implications of these changes.

Social determinants of health (SDOH), non-medical factors that affect health outcomes, are another area of heightened awareness, concern, and research by neuroscience nurses. These factors are important in identifying and addressing the health inequities that affect persons with neurologic conditions. Neuroscience nurses in all settings help patients and families with neurologic conditions identify correct information and discern disinformation due to the vast array of content on social media platforms (Villaruel & James, 2022).

While the SDOH are addressed in many ways by all nurses, one example of a health inequity of particular concern to neuroscience nurses is the high incidence of early-onset stroke and poorer outcomes in African Americans compared to other racial groups. Therefore, a stroke counseling intervention was developed for adult African Americans. While still not fully tested and implemented, this age, culture, and gender-focused intervention has great promise for reducing the risk of stroke in young African American adults (Aycock et al., 2023).

Complementary and alternative medicine (CAM) options are further expanding care. Neuroscience nurses are challenged to keep abreast of CAM developments and integrative health strategies and institute practices that guide individuals in their use. Nursing interactions are moving beyond traditional settings into novel areas such as industry, legal practice, insurance, government, media, and social service areas. Neuroscience nurses are encouraged to explore new venues that utilize their expertise.

The healthcare industry is challenged to optimize patient safety, patient and practitioner satisfaction, patient outcomes, and healthcare organization profitability. Patient safety will remain at the forefront of neuroscience nursing practice. The value of neuroscience nurses in patient safety and positive patient outcomes in hospital settings is well demonstrated (Drollinger & Prasun, 2023). Employers are addressing workplace problems to retain nurses. Safe patient handling, shift and scheduling options, integration of technological support into practice, and alternative roles in the healthcare setting have enabled nurses to remain in the workplace.

A changing healthcare delivery system has a major impact on the neuroscience nurse's scope of practice. Societal, economic, and political pressures are driving the development of less costly means to meet public healthcare needs. One way neuroscience nurses can be intimately involved in this process is by using neuroscience APRNs to deliver care. Neuroscience APRNs, with their expanded knowledge base and expertise, can provide high-quality care in a more cost-effective manner than a traditional medical model (Holleman et al., 2010; Mills et al., 1999). One example of this is a nurse practitioner-led pediatric baclofen pump program to reduce risk of baclofen withdrawal and address common troubleshooting issues (Buxton et al., 2017). Neuroscience APRNs can also function as consultants to registered nurses and other healthcare team members. Collaboration, effective use of resources, cost-containment, increased patient participation, timely goal achievement, and continuity of care are concepts critical to the future of neuroscience nursing and healthcare systems as a whole.

The changing healthcare market will also impact the practice of neuroscience nursing. As the United States population ages, chronic illness will predominate, and a shift in care delivery from acute to chronic illness will be necessary. Neuroscience nurses are challenged to redirect their practice, and educators are challenged to meet the demand for practitioners. The focus of healthcare providers is evolving to address prevention and problem management across the lifespan, rather than focusing on episodic care alone.

The need for healthcare reform is a major concern. A reformed healthcare system focused on primary care, prevention, and chronic disease management can help alleviate the financial and social costs of treating preventable and chronic diseases. Interprofessional teams and care coordination across the illness trajectory will be key components in the new system, arenas in which neuroscience nurses are familiar and have demonstrated their value.

Neuroscience nurses are positioned to play key roles in reforming and restructuring care delivery systems. A major shift from inpatient to outpatient care settings continues to occur. Expanded roles in community-based programs are developing. Neuroscience nurses are encouraged to support and participate in the medical or healthcare home model for care management. Neuroscience APRNs should also be utilized to the full extent of their scope of practice, consistent with education and competencies.

When neuroscience APRNs are utilized to the full extent of their scope of practice, patient outcomes are improved. An example of this is the implementation of an APRN-led clinic for patients after acute care discharge following an ischemic stroke. This project led to the time to follow up for patients being decreased from approximately 4 months to 1 month after acute care discharge. Timely follow-up after discharge for this population can reduce unnecessary 30-day readmission rates (Mitchell et al., 2022).

As healthcare evolves, nurses may experience greater opportunities to function within their full scope of practice across various settings. A reformed healthcare system will provide incentives and financial support to utilize nurses in various roles, promote a full scope of practice, and eliminate the current payment practices that create barriers to innovative and effective models of practice and care delivery (National Academy of Medicine, 2021).

Nursing, as a profession, continues to face dilemmas in entry into practice, the autonomy of advanced practice, continued competence, multistate licensure, and the appropriate educational credentials for professional certification. Neuroscience nurses have a professional responsibility to maintain competence in their practice area. Employers who provide opportunities for professional development and continuing education promote a positive practice environment in which nurses can maintain and enhance skills and competencies. The ability to recruit an adequate number of nurses to the specialty, as well as retain those who are currently practicing, is critical to the future of neuroscience nursing.

Technology offers a better work environment for neuroscience nurses when designed and implemented in a manner that supports nurses' work. These work environments can include conventional locations—hospitals, clinics, and patient homes—as well as virtual spaces such as online discussion groups, email, interactive video, and virtual interaction. Ideally, technology eliminates redundancy and duplication of documentation, reduces errors, removes interruptions for missing supplies, equipment, and medications, and eases access to data, thereby allowing the neuroscience nurse more time with the healthcare consumer (IOM, 2009). Technology use, however, is not without risk, and demands diligence by neuroscience nurses to consider the impact on the scope of neuroscience nursing practice and the ethical implications for healthcare consumers as well as the nurse.

Regardless of practice venue, over the next decade, neuroscience nurses will continue to partner with others to advance the nation's health through collaborative initiatives. As practice changes evolve, neuroscience nurses are at the forefront to address these challenges The primary responsibility of neuroscience nursing will remain the realm of human responses to actual or potential health problems secondary to nervous system conditions.

SUMMARY OF THE SCOPE OF NEUROSCIENCE NURSING PRACTICE

The dynamic nature of the healthcare practice environment and the growing body of nursing clinical science provide both the impetus and the opportunity for nursing to ensure competent nursing practice in all settings for all healthcare consumers, and to promote ongoing professional development that enhances the quality of nursing practice. *Neuroscience Nursing: Scope and Standards of Practice, Fourth Edition* assists that process by delineating the professional scope and standards and responsibilities of all professional neuroscience nurses, regardless of setting. As such, it can serve as a basis for

- Position recruitment announcement;
- Position description creation;
- New employee orientation;
- Performance appraisal and evaluation;
- Agency policy, protocol, and procedure development;
- Competency identification and development;
- Educating individuals regarding the role of neuroscience nurses;
- Quality improvement systems and program evaluation efforts;

- Development and evaluation of school nursing service delivery systems and organizational structures;
- Educational offerings;
- Database development, data collection, and research;
- Establishing a legal standard;
- Healthcare reimbursement and financing methodologies; and
- Regulatory review and revision.

Standards of Practice for Neuroscience Nursing Practice

STANDARDS OF PRACTICE FOR NEUROSCIENCE NURSING

Standard 1. Assessment

The neuroscience nurse collects pertinent data and information relative to the healthcare consumer's health or the situation.

COMPETENCIES

The neuroscience nurse

- Creates the safest environment possible for conducting assessments;
- Collects pertinent data related to health and quality of life in a systematic, ongoing manner, with compassion and respect for the wholeness, inherent dignity, worth, and unique attributes of every person, including but not limited to demographics, environmental and occupational exposures, social determinants of health, health disparities, and physical, functional, psychosocial, emotional, cognitive, spiritual or transpersonal, sexual, sociocultural, age-related, environmental, or lifestyle or economic assessments (see Standard 9);
- Utilizes a health and wellness model of assessment that incorporates integrative approaches to data collection and honors the whole person;

- Recognizes the healthcare consumer or designated person as the decision-maker regarding their own health by honoring their care preferences;
- Explores the healthcare consumer's culture, values, preferences, expressed and unexpressed needs, and knowledge of the healthcare situation (see Standard 9);
- Assesses the impact of family dynamics on the healthcare consumer's health and wellness;
- Identifies enhancements and barriers to effective communication based on personal, cognitive, psychosocial, literacy, financial, and cultural considerations (see Standard 10);
- Engages the healthcare consumer, family, significant others, and interprofessional team members in holistic, culturally sensitive data collection;
- Integrates knowledge from current local, regional, national, and global health initiatives and environmental factors into the assessment process:
  - State and local departments of health
  - World Health Organization: who.int/
  - World Health Organization Health topics: who.int/ health-topics/
  - Healthy People: healthy-people.gov/
  - Centers for Disease Control and Prevention: cdc.gov/nchs/nhis/ dex.htmdex.htm
- Prioritizes data collection based on the healthcare consumer's immediate condition, the anticipated needs of the healthcare consumer or situation, or both;
- Uses evidence-based assessment techniques, as well as available data and information to identify patterns and variances in the consumer's health;
- Remains knowledgeable about constantly changing technologies that impact the assessment process (e.g., telehealth and artificial intelligence);
- Analyzes assessment data to identify patterns, trends, and situations that impact the person's health and wellness;

- Validates the analysis with the healthcare consumer;
- Documents data accurately and makes accessible to the interprofessional team in a timely manner;
- Communicates changes in person's condition to the interprofessional team;
- Applies the provisions of the ANA *Code of Ethics*, legal standards, guidelines, and policies to the collection, maintenance, use, and dissemination of data and information; and
- Recognizes the impact of one's own personal attitudes, values, beliefs, and biases on the assessment process (see Standards 7, 9, and 15).

Additional Competencies for the Graduate-Level Prepared Neuroscience RN

In addition to the neuroscience nurse competencies, the graduate-level prepared neuroscience RN

- Uses advanced knowledge, skills, and assessment techniques and approaches to maintain, enhance, and improve health;
- Analyzes the effect of interactions among individuals, family, community, and social systems on health and illness; and
- Synthesizes the results and information leading to clinical understanding.

Additional Competencies for the Neuroscience APRN

In addition to the competencies of the neuroscience registered nurse and the graduate-level prepared neuroscience RN, the neuroscience APRN

- Initiates diagnostic tests and procedures relevant to the healthcare consumer's ongoing health status, and
- Uses advanced knowledge, skills, assessment techniques and approaches within identified population foci to maintain, enhance, and improve health.

Standard 2. Diagnosis

The neuroscience nurse analyzes assessment data to determine actual or potential diagnoses, problems, and issues.

COMPETENCIES

The neuroscience nurse

- Identifies actual or potential risks to the healthcare consumer's health and safety or barriers to health which may include but are not limited to interpersonal, systematic, cultural, socioeconomic, or environmental circumstances;
- Uses assessment data, standardized classification systems, technology, and clinical decision support tools to articulate actual or potential diagnoses, problems, and issues;
- Identifies the healthcare consumer's strengths and abilities, including but not limited to support systems, health literacy, and engagement in self-care;
- Verifies the diagnoses, problems, and issues with the healthcare consumer and interprofessional colleagues;
- Prioritizes diagnoses, problems, and issues based on mutually established goals to meet the needs of the healthcare consumer across the health-illness continuum and the care continuum; and
- Documents diagnoses, problems, strengths, and issues in a manner that facilitates the development of the expected outcomes and collaborative plan.

ADDITIONAL COMPETENCIES FOR THE GRADUATE-LEVEL PREPARED NEUROSCIENCE RN

In addition to the neuroscience nurse competencies, the graduate-level prepared neuroscience RN

- Uses information and communication technologies to analyze diagnostic practice patterns of nurses and other members of the interprofessional healthcare team, and

- Employs aggregate-level data to articulate diagnoses, problems, and issues of healthcare consumers, and organizational systems.

ADDITIONAL COMPETENCIES FOR THE NEUROSCIENCE APRN

In addition to the competencies of the neuroscience registered nurse and the graduate-level prepared neuroscience RN, the neuroscience APRN

- Formulates differential diagnoses based on assessment, history, physical examination, and diagnostic test results, and
- Incorporates standard terminologies and coding methodologies to ensure correct documentation of identified diagnoses.

Standard 3. Outcomes Identification

The neuroscience nurse identifies expected outcomes for a plan individualized to the healthcare consumer or the situation.

COMPETENCIES

The neuroscience nurse

- Engages the healthcare consumer, interprofessional team, and others in partnership to identify expected outcomes and expected time frames;
- Collaborates with the healthcare consumer to formulate culturally sensitive expected outcomes derived from assessments and diagnoses;
- Uses clinical expertise and current evidence-based practice to identify health risks, benefits, costs, and expected trajectory of the condition;
- Collaborates with the healthcare consumer to define expected outcomes that integrate the healthcare consumer's culture, values, and ethical considerations;
- Generates a time frame for the attainment of expected outcomes;
- Develops expected outcomes that facilitate coordination of care;

- Utilizes assessment and diagnosis to formulate expected outcomes;
- Modifies expected outcomes based on the evaluation of the status of the healthcare consumer and situation;
- Documents outcomes as measurable goals; and
- Evaluates the actual outcomes in relation to expected outcomes, safety, and quality standards.

Additional Competencies for the Graduate-Level Prepared Neuroscience RN, Including the Neuroscience APRN

In addition to the competencies of the neuroscience nurse, the graduate-level prepared neuroscience RN, including the neuroscience APRN

- Defines expected outcomes that incorporate cost and clinical effectiveness and are aligned with the outcomes identified by members of the interprofessional team;
- Differentiates outcomes that require care process interventions from those that require system-level actions;
- Integrates scientific evidence and best practices to achieve expected outcomes;
- Advocates for outcomes that reflect the healthcare consumer's culture, values, and ethical concerns;
- Actively leads the education of the healthcare consumer and interdisciplinary team regarding the identification of and achievement of anticipated expected outcomes; and
- Identifies quality outcome measures in relation to expected outcomes, safety, and quality standards.

Standard 4. Planning

The neuroscience nurse develops a collaborative plan encompassing strategies to achieve expected outcomes.

Competencies

The neuroscience nurse
- Develops an individualized, holistic, evidence-based plan in partnership with the healthcare consumer, family, significant others, and interprofessional team;

- Designs innovative nursing practices that can be incorporated into the plan;
- Prioritizes elements of the plan based on the assessment of the healthcare consumer's level of safety needs to include risks, benefits, and alternatives;
- Establishes the plan priorities with the healthcare consumer, family, significant others, and interprofessional team;
- Advocates for compassionate, responsible, and appropriate use of interventions to minimize unwarranted or unwanted treatment, healthcare consumer suffering, or both;
- Includes strategies in the plan that address each of the identified diagnoses, problems or issues. These strategies may include but are not limited to
  - Maintaining health and wellness;
  - Promotion of comfort;
  - Promotion of wholeness, growth, and development;
  - Promotion and restoration of health and wellness;
  - Prevention of illness, injury, disease, complications, and trauma;
  - Alleviation of suffering;
  - Supportive care; and
  - Mitigation of environmental or occupational risks
- Incorporates an implementation pathway that describes a timeline, steps, and milestones;
- Provides for the coordination and continuity of care;
- Identifies cost and economic implications of the plan;
- Develops a plan that reflects compliance with current statutes, rules and regulations, and standards;
- Modifies the plan according to the ongoing assessment of the healthcare consumer's response and other outcome indicators;
- Documents the plan in a manner that uses standardized language or recognized terminology; and
- Actively contributes at all levels to the development and continuous improvement of systems that support the planning process.

ADDITIONAL COMPETENCIES FOR THE GRADUATE-LEVEL PREPARED NEUROSCIENCE RN

In addition to the neuroscience nurse competencies, the graduate-level prepared neuroscience RN

- Designs strategies and approaches to meet the complex health needs of healthcare consumers;
- Develops interprofessional processes to address the identified diagnoses, health challenges, problems, issues, or opportunities in partnership with the healthcare consumer, family, and significant others; and
- Leads the design and development of interprofessional processes to address the identified diagnoses, health challenges, and issues or opportunities.

ADDITIONAL COMPETENCIES FOR THE NEUROSCIENCE APRN

In addition to the neuroscience nurse competencies and the graduate-level prepared neuroscience RN competencies, the neuroscience APRN integrates assessment strategies, consultative and diagnostic strategies, and therapeutic interventions that reflect evidence-based advanced knowledge and practice within the neuroscience population.

Standard 5. Implementation

The neuroscience nurse implements the identified plan.

COMPETENCIES

The neuroscience nurse

- Demonstrates caring behaviors to develop therapeutic relationships;
- Provides care that focuses on the healthcare consumer;
- Advocates for the needs of diverse populations across the life span;

- Uses critical thinking and technology solutions to implement the nursing process by collecting, measuring, recording, retrieving, trending, and analyzing data and information to enhance healthcare consumer outcomes and nursing practice;
- Partners with the healthcare consumer to implement the plan in a safe, effective, efficient, timely, and equitable manner;
- Engages interprofessional team partners in implementation of the plan through collaboration and communication across the continuum of care;
- Uses evidence-based interventions and strategies to achieve mutually identified goals and outcomes specific to the problem or needs;
- Delegates according to the health, safety, and welfare of the healthcare consumer;
- Delegates after considering the circumstance, person, task, direction or communication, supervision, evaluation, as well as the state nurse practice act regulations, institution, and regulatory entities while maintaining accountability for the care; and
- Documents implementation and any modifications, including changes or omissions, of the identified plan.

ADDITIONAL COMPETENCIES FOR THE
GRADUATE-LEVEL PREPARED NEUROSCIENCE RN

In addition to the neuroscience nurse competencies, the graduate-level prepared neuroscience RN

- Translates evidence-based findings into practice;
- Demonstrates ethical and critical decision-making, effective working relationships, and a systems perspective;
- Uses theory-driven approaches to effect organizational or system change;
- Applies quality principles while articulating methods, tools, performance measures, and standards as they relate to implementation of the plan;

- Uses systems, organizations, and community resources to lead effective change and implement the plan;
- Leads interprofessional teams to effectively communicate and collaborate; and
- Serves as a consultant to provide additional insight and potential solutions.

Additional Competencies for the Neuroscience APRN

In addition to the neuroscience nurse competencies and the graduate-level prepared neuroscience RN, the neuroscience APRN

- Uses prescriptive authority, procedures, referrals, treatments, and therapies in accordance with state and federal laws and regulations;
- Prescribes traditional and integrative evidence-based treatments, therapies, and procedures that are compatible with the healthcare consumer's cultural preferences, norms, and abilities;
- Prescribes evidence-based pharmacological agents and treatments according to clinical indicators and results of diagnostic and laboratory tests; and
- Provides clinical consultation for healthcare consumers and professionals to improve care and outcomes.

Standard 5A. Coordination of Care

The neuroscience nurse coordinates care delivery.

Competencies

The neuroscience nurse

- Collaborates with the healthcare consumer and the interprofessional team to help manage healthcare based on mutually agreed-upon outcomes;
- Organizes the components of the plan with input from the healthcare consumer and other stakeholders;

- Manages the healthcare consumer's care to reach mutually agreed-upon outcomes;
- Engages healthcare consumers in self-care to achieve preferred goals for quality of life;
- Assists the healthcare consumer to identify options for care and navigate the healthcare system and its services;
- Communicates with the healthcare consumer, interprofessional team, and community-based resources to effect safe transitions in continuity of care;
- Advocates for the delivery of dignified and person-centered care by the interprofessional team; and
- Documents the coordination of care.

ADDITIONAL COMPETENCIES FOR THE GRADUATE-LEVEL PREPARED NEUROSCIENCE RN

In addition to the neuroscience nurse competencies, the graduate-level prepared neuroscience RN

- Provides leadership in the coordination of interprofessional healthcare for the delivery of integrated system-level healthcare consumer services to achieve safe, efficient, timely, person-centered, and equitable care, and
- Manages identified healthcare consumer panels or populations.

ADDITIONAL COMPETENCIES FOR THE NEUROSCIENCE APRN

In addition to the neuroscience nurse competencies and the graduate-level prepared neuroscience RN, the neuroscience APRN

- Synthesizes data and information to prescribe and provide necessary system and community support measures, including modifications of environments, and
- Serves as the healthcare consumer's provider to coordinate healthcare services in accordance with state and federal laws and regulations.

Standard 5B. Health Teaching and Health Promotion

The neuroscience nurse employs strategies to teach and promote health and wellness.

COMPETENCIES

The neuroscience nurse

- Provides opportunities for the healthcare consumer to identify needed health promotion, disease prevention, and self-management topics such as healthy lifestyles, self-care and risk management, coping, adaptability, and resiliency;
- Uses health promotion and health teaching methods in collaboration with the healthcare consumer's values, beliefs, health practices, developmental level, learning needs, readiness and ability to learn, language preference, spirituality, culture, and socioeconomic status;
- Uses feedback from the healthcare consumer and other assessments to determine the effectiveness of the employed strategies;
- Uses technologies to communicate health promotion and disease prevention information to the healthcare consumer;
- Provides healthcare consumers with information and education about intended effects and potential adverse effects of the plan of care;
- Engages consumer alliance and advocacy groups in health teaching and health promotion activities for healthcare consumers; and
- Provides anticipatory guidance to healthcare consumers to promote health and prevent or reduce risk.

ADDITIONAL COMPETENCIES FOR THE GRADUATE-LEVEL PREPARED NEUROSCIENCE RN, INCLUDING THE NEUROSCIENCE APRN

In addition to the competencies of the neuroscience nurse, the graduate-level prepared neuroscience RN, including the neuroscience APRN

- Synthesizes evidence on risk behaviors, gender roles, learning theories, behavioral change theories, motivational theories, translational theories for evidence-based practice, epidemiology, and other related theories and frameworks when designing health education information, tools, and programs; and
- Evaluates health information resources for applicability, accuracy, readability, and comprehensibility to help healthcare consumers access quality health information.

Standard 6. Evaluation

The neuroscience nurse evaluates the progress toward attainment of goals and outcomes.

COMPETENCIES

The neuroscience nurse

- Uses applicable standards and defined criteria (e.g., Quality and Safety Education for Nurses [QSEN], Quadruple Aim, and the Institute for Healthcare Improvement [IHI]);
- Conducts a systematic, ongoing, and criteria-based evaluation of the outcomes in relation to the structures, processes, and timeline prescribed in the plan;
- Collaborates with the healthcare consumer and others involved in the care or situation in the evaluation process;
- Determines, in partnership with the healthcare consumer and other stakeholders, the patient-centeredness, effectiveness, efficiency, safety, timeliness, and equitability of the strategies in relation to the responses to the plan and the attainment of the outcomes—other defined criteria (e.g., QSEN) may be used as well;
- Uses ongoing assessment data, other data and information resources and benchmarks, research, and meta-analysis for the analytic activities to revise the diagnoses, outcomes, plan, implementation, and evaluation strategies as needed;
- Documents the results of the evaluation;

- Reports evaluation data in a timely fashion; and
- Shares evaluation data and conclusions with the healthcare consumer and other stakeholders to promote clarity and transparency in accordance with state, federal, organizational, and professional requirements.

ADDITIONAL COMPETENCIES FOR THE GRADUATE-LEVEL PREPARED NEUROSCIENCE RN, INCLUDING THE NEUROSCIENCE APRN

In addition to the competencies of the neuroscience registered nurse, the graduate-level prepared neuroscience RN, including the neuroscience APRN

- Synthesizes evaluation data to determine the plan's impact on the consumer and population health, and
- Uses the results of the evaluation to recommend and conduct research, process, policy, procedure, or protocol revisions when warranted.

STANDARDS OF PROFESSIONAL PERFORMANCE FOR NEUROSCIENCE NURSING

Standard 7. Ethics

The neuroscience nurse integrates ethics in all aspects of practice.

COMPETENCIES

The neuroscience nurse

- Integrates the *Code of Ethics for Nurses with Interpretive Statements* (ANA, 2015) as a moral foundation to guide nursing practice and decision making;
- Demonstrates that every person is worthy of nursing care through the provisions of respectful, person-centered, compassionate care, regardless of personal history or characteristics (beneficence);

- Advocates for healthcare consumer perspectives, preferences, and rights to informed decision-making and self-determination (respect for autonomy);
- Demonstrates a primary commitment to the recipients of healthcare services in all settings and situations (fidelity);
- Acts to prevent breaches to privacy and confidentiality;
- Safeguards sensitive information within ethical, legal, and regulatory parameters (non-maleficence);
- Identifies ethics resources within the practice setting to assist and collaborate in addressing ethical issues;
- Integrates principles of social justice in all aspects of nursing practice (justice);
- Refines ethical competence through continued personal and professional development;
- Depicts one's professional nursing identity through demonstrated values and ethics, knowledge, leadership, and professional comportment;
- Engages in self-care and self-reflection practices to support and preserve personal health, well-being, and integrity;
- Contributes to the establishment and maintenance of an ethical environment that is conducive to safe, quality healthcare;
- Collaborates with other professionals and the public to protect human rights, promote health diplomacy, enhance cultural sensitivity and congruence, and reduce health disparities; and
- Represents the nursing perspective in clinic, institutional, community, or professional association ethics discussions.

ADDITIONAL COMPETENCIES FOR THE GRADUATE-LEVEL PREPARED NEUROSCIENCE RN, INCLUDING THE NEUROSCIENCE APRN

In addition to the competencies of the registered nurse, the graduate-level prepared neuroscience RN, including the neuroscience APRN

- Demonstrates advanced knowledge of ethical analyses, ethical principles of respect for autonomy, beneficence, non-maleficence, and justice, and their relationship to ethical nursing practice;

- Acts as an educational resource by providing leadership in developing nurses' ethical competence, including ethical decision-making, to address emerging or recurrent ethical issues;
- Creates open moral spaces conducive to interprofessional ethical dialogue;
- Mediates ethical conflicts acting as a liaison among individuals, family, and the healthcare team;
- Advances ethics knowledge and practice through scholarly inquiry, professional standards development, and policy generation; and
- Represents the profession as a subject matter expert, advisor, or consultant, locally, statewide, regionally, nationally and internationally.

Standard 8. Advocacy

The neuroscience nurse demonstrates advocacy in all roles and settings.

COMPETENCIES

The neuroscience nurse

- Champions the voice of the healthcare consumer;
- Recommends appropriate levels of care, timely and appropriate transitions, and allocation of resources to optimize outcomes;
- Promotes safe care of healthcare consumers, safe work environments, and sufficient resources;
- Participates in healthcare initiatives on behalf of the healthcare consumer and the system(s) where neuroscience nursing happens;
- Demonstrates a willingness to address persistent, pervasive systemic issues;
- Informs the political arena about the role of neuroscience nurses and the vital components necessary for neuroscience nurses to provide optimal care delivery;

- Empowers all members of the healthcare team to include the healthcare consumer in care decisions, including limitation of treatment and end of life;
- Embraces diversity, equity, inclusivity, health promotion, and healthcare for individuals of diverse geographic, cultural, ethnic, racial, gender, and spiritual backgrounds across the life span;
- Develops policies that improve care delivery and access for underserved and vulnerable populations;
- Promotes policies, regulations, and legislation at the local, state, and national level to improve healthcare access and delivery of healthcare;
- Considers societal, political, economic, and cultural factors to address social determinants of health;
- Role models advocacy behavior;
- Addresses the urgent need for a diverse and inclusive workforce as a strategy to improve outcomes related to the social determinants of health and inequities in the healthcare system;
- Advances policies, programs, and practices within the healthcare environment that maintain, sustain, and restore the environment and natural world; and
- Contributes to professional organizations, including the AANN.

ADDITIONAL COMPETENCIES FOR THE GRADUATE-LEVEL PREPARED NEUROSCIENCE RN

In addition to the competencies of the neuroscience registered nurse, the graduate-level prepared neuroscience RN

- Analyzes the impact of geographic, societal, political, economic, and cultural factors on healthcare disparities;
- Develops alliances with various groups to promote advocacy goals;
- Pursues resources to improve the delivery of care services and outcomes; and

- Influences leaders, legislators, governmental agencies, nongovernmental organizations, and international bodies to address determinants of health.

ADDITIONAL COMPETENCIES FOR THE NEUROSCIENCE APRN

In addition to the competencies of the neuroscience nurse, and the graduate-level prepared neuroscience RN, the neuroscience APRN

- Promotes universal application of full practice authority in all settings and roles to meet healthcare needs of diverse neuroscience populations;
- Advocates for a direct reporting structure to the appropriate advanced practice nursing leadership position;
- Endorses the profession's *Consensus Model for APRN Regulation: Licensure, Accreditation, Certification, & Education*;
- Maintains safety and culturally based integrity within neuroscience APRN practices; and
- Fosters a just culture within neuroscience APRN practices.

Standard 9. Respectful and Equitable Practice

The neuroscience nurse practices with cultural humility and inclusiveness.

COMPETENCIES

The neuroscience nurse

- Demonstrates respect, equity, and empathy in actions and interactions with all healthcare consumers;
- Respects consumer decisions without bias;
- Participates in life-long learning to understand cultural preferences, worldviews, choices, and decision-making processes of diverse consumers;
- Reflects upon personal and cultural values, beliefs, biases, and heritage;
- Applies knowledge of differences in health beliefs, practices, and communication patterns without assigning value to the differences;

- Addresses the effects and impact of discrimination and oppression on practice within and among diverse groups;
- Uses appropriate skills and tools for the culture, literacy, and language of the individuals and population served;
- Communicates with appropriate language and behaviors, including the use of qualified healthcare interpreters and translators in accordance with consumer needs and preferences;
- Serves as a role model and educator for cultural humility and the recognition and appreciation of diversity and inclusivity;
- Identifies the cultural-specific meaning of interactions, terms, and content;
- Advocates for policies that promote health and prevent harm among diverse healthcare consumers and groups;
- Promotes equity in all aspects of health and healthcare; and
- Advances organizational policies, programs, services, and practices that reflect respect, equity, and values for diversity and inclusion.

ADDITIONAL COMPETENCIES FOR THE GRADUATE-LEVEL PREPARED NEUROSCIENCE RN, INCLUDING THE NEUROSCIENCE APRN

In addition to the competencies of the registered nurse, the graduate-level prepared neuroscience RN, including the neuroscience APRN

- Engages consumers, key stakeholders, and others in designing and establishing internal and external cross-cultural partnerships;
- Conducts research and quality improvement initiatives to improve healthcare and healthcare outcomes for culturally diverse consumers;
- Develops recruitment and retention strategies to achieve a multicultural workforce; and
- Promotes shared decision-making solutions in planning and evaluating processes when the healthcare consumer's cultural preferences and norms may create incompatibility with evidence-based practice.

Standard 10. Communication

The neuroscience nurse communicates effectively in all areas of professional practice.

COMPETENCIES

The neuroscience nurse

- Assesses their own communication skills and effectiveness;
- Demonstrates cultural humility, equity, and respect when communicating;
- Assesses communication ability, health literacy, resources, and preferences of healthcare consumers to inform the interprofessional team and others;
- Uses language translation resources to ensure effective communication;
- Incorporates appropriate alternative strategies to communicate effectively with healthcare consumers who have cognitive, visual, speech, language, or communication difficulties;
- Uses communication styles and methods that demonstrate professionalism, caring, respect, active listening, authenticity, and trust;
- Conveys accurate information to individuals, families, and members of the interprofessional team;
- Clarifies and validates understanding of the rationale for care processes and decisions with individuals, families, and members of the interprofessional team;
- Verbalizes the preferences and choices of the patient and family when care process and decisions do not appear to be in the best interest of the patient and family;
- Maintains communication with interprofessional team members and others to facilitate safe transitions and continuity in care delivery;
- Contributes the nursing perspective in interactions with others and discussions with the interprofessional team using closed loop communication;

- Uses appropriate resources to disclose concerns related to potential
  or actual hazards or deviations from the standard of care;
- Demonstrates and solicits feedback for continuous improvement
  of communication and conflict resolution skills; and
- Advocates for escalation of care when patient needs are not
  adequately met.

ADDITIONAL COMPETENCIES FOR THE GRADUATE-LEVEL PREPARED NEUROSCIENCE RN, INCLUDING THE NEUROSCIENCE APRN

In addition to the competencies of the neuroscience nurse, the graduate-level prepared neuroscience RN, including the neuroscience APRN, leads in creating environments that promote and sustain effective and ongoing communication.

Standard 11. Collaboration

The neuroscience nurse collaborates with the healthcare consumer and other key stakeholders.

COMPETENCIES

The neuroscience nurse

- Partners with the healthcare consumer and key stakeholders to
  advocate for and affect change, leading to positive outcomes and
  quality care;
- Treats others with dignity and respect in all interactions;
- Uses the unique and complementary abilities of all members of the
  interprofessional team to optimize attainment of desired outcomes;
- Articulates the neuroscience nurse's role and responsibilities
  within the interprofessional team;
- Uses appropriate tools and techniques, including information systems
  and technologies, to facilitate discussion and team functions in a
  manner that protects dignity, respect, privacy, and confidentiality;
- Promotes engagement through consensus building and conflict
  management;

- Uses effective group dynamics and strategies to enhance team performance of the interprofessional team;
- Partners with all stakeholders to create, implement, and evaluate a comprehensive neuroscience plan; and
- Role models the development of shared goals, clear roles, mutual trust, effective communication, efficient processes, and measurable outcomes within the interprofessional team.

ADDITIONAL COMPETENCIES FOR THE GRADUATE-LEVEL PREPARED NEUROSCIENCE RN, INCLUDING THE NEUROSCIENCE APRN

In addition to the competencies of the neuroscience nurse, the graduate-level prepared neuroscience RN, including the neuroscience APRN

- Participates in interprofessional activities, including but not limited to education, consultation, management, technological development, and research to enhance neuroscience outcomes;
- Leads in establishing, improving, and sustaining collaborative relationships to achieve safe, quality care for healthcare consumers;
- Advances interprofessional plan-of-care documentation and communication, rationales for plan-of-care changes, and collaborative discussions to improve healthcare consumer outcomes; and
- Leads high-performing interprofessional teams in response to situational needs of healthcare consumers.

Standard 12. Leadership

The neuroscience nurse leads within the profession and practice setting.

COMPETENCIES

The neuroscience nurse
- Promotes effective relationships (relational coordination) to achieve quality outcomes and a culture of safety;
- Leads decision-making groups;

- Embraces practice innovations and role performance to achieve lifelong personal and professional goals;
- Communicates to lead change, influence others, and resolve conflict;
- Mentors colleagues and others to enhance their knowledge, skills, and abilities;
- Implements evidence-based practices for safe, quality healthcare and healthcare consumer satisfaction;
- Engages in creating an environment that promotes respect, trust, and integrity;
- Demonstrates authority, ownership, accountability, and responsibility for appropriate delegation of nursing care;
- Participates in professional activities and organizations for professional growth and influence; and
- Advocates for all aspects of human and environmental health in practice and policy.

ADDITIONAL COMPETENCIES FOR THE GRADUATE-LEVEL PREPARED NEUROSCIENCE RN, INCLUDING THE NEUROSCIENCE APRN

In addition to the neuroscience registered nurse competencies, the graduate-level prepared neuroscience RN, including the neuroscience APRN

- Engages with decision-making bodies to implement an effective interprofessional environment that improves healthcare consumer outcomes and satisfaction;
- Interprets advanced practice nursing roles for policymakers and healthcare consumers;
- Models expert nursing practice to interprofessional team members and healthcare consumers; and
- Mentors colleagues in their professional growth and participation in succession planning.

Standard 13. Education

The neuroscience nurse seeks knowledge and competence that reflects current nursing practice and promotes futuristic thinking.

The neuroscience nurse

- Identifies learning needs based on nursing knowledge, the various roles the nurse may assume, and changing population-specific needs;
- Participates in ongoing professional development activities related to nursing and interprofessional knowledge bases and professional topics;
- Mentors nurses who are new to their roles for the purpose of ensuring successful enculturation, orientation, competence, and emotional support;
- Supports acculturation of nurses new to their roles by role modeling, encouraging, advocating, and sharing information relative to optimal care delivery;
- Mentors peers in role and practice;
- Demonstrates a commitment to lifelong learning through critical thinking, self-reflection, inquiry for learning, and personal growth;
- Seeks experiences that reflect current practice to develop, maintain, and advance knowledge, skills, human functioning, attitudes, and judgment in clinical practice or role performance;
- Acquires knowledge and skills relative to the role, population, specialty, setting, and global or local health situation;
- Participates in and advocates through formal consultations or informal discussions to address issues in nursing practice as an application of education and knowledge (see Standard 8);
- Identifies modifications or accommodations needed to deliver education based on the learner's needs;
- Shares educational findings, experiences, and ideas with peers and interprofessional colleagues;
- Facilitates a work environment supportive to the ongoing education of healthcare professionals and interprofessional colleagues;

- Maintains a professional portfolio that provides evidence of individual competence and lifelong learning; and
- Seeks and maintains neuroscience nursing certification.

ADDITIONAL COMPETENCIES FOR THE GRADUATE-LEVEL PREPARED NEUROSCIENCE RN, INCLUDING THE NEUROSCIENCE APRN

In addition to the competencies of the neuroscience nurse, the graduate-level prepared neuroscience RN, including the neuroscience APRN

- Uses current healthcare research findings and other evidence to expand clinical knowledge, skills, human functioning, and judgment, to enhance role performance, and to increase knowledge of professional issues;
- Analyzes issues, trends, and supporting data to determine and address the educational needs of individuals, organizations, communities; and
- Promotes the development of sustainable local, system-wide, or global programs and initiatives that facilitate professional role competence and growth.

Standard 14. Scholarly Inquiry

The neuroscience nurse integrates scholarship, evidence, and research findings into practice.

COMPETENCIES

The neuroscience nurse

- Identifies questions in the healthcare or practice setting that can be answered by scholarly inquiry;
- Uses current evidence-based knowledge, combined with clinical expertise and healthcare consumer values and preferences, to guide practice in all settings;

- Participates in the formulation of evidence-based practice;
- Uses evidence to expand knowledge, skills, human functioning, and judgment to enhance role performance and to increase knowledge of professional issues for themselves and others;
- Shares peer-reviewed, evidence-based findings with colleagues to integrate knowledge into nursing practice;
- Incorporates evidence and nursing research when initiating changes and improving quality in nursing practice;
- Articulates the value of research and scholarly inquiry and their application to one's practice and healthcare setting;
- Promotes ethical principles of research in practice and the healthcare setting; and
- Reviews nursing research for application in practice and the healthcare setting.

ADDITIONAL COMPETENCIES FOR THE GRADUATE-LEVEL PREPARED NEUROSCIENCE RN, INCLUDING THE NEUROSCIENCE APRN

In addition to the neuroscience nurse competencies, the graduate-level prepared neuroscience RN, including the neuroscience APRN

- Uses critical thinking skills to connect theory and research to practice;
- Critically appraises data and information to generate meaningful evidence for nursing practice;
- Generates knowledge by conducting or synthesizing research and other evidence that examines and evaluates current practice, knowledge, theories, criteria, and innovative approaches to contribute to quality outcomes;
- Translates evidence-based knowledge in all settings;
- Implements evidence-based knowledge to improve organizational structures and systems;
- Advocates for the ethical conduct of translational and other research with particular attention to the protection of the healthcare consumer as a research participant;

- Promotes a climate of collaborative research and scholarly inquiry;
- Mentors other nurses to develop scholarly inquiry skills; and
- Disseminates scholarly findings through activities such as presentations, publications, consultation, and journal clubs.

Standard 15. Quality of Practice

The neuroscience nurse contributes to quality nursing practice.

COMPETENCIES

The neuroscience nurse

- Ensures that nursing practice is safe, effective, efficient, equitable, timely, and patient-centered;
- Incorporates evidence into nursing practice to optimize outcomes;
- Identifies barriers and opportunities to improve healthcare safety, effectiveness, efficiency, equitability, timeliness, and patient-centeredness;
- Recommends strategies to improve nursing practice quality;
- Uses creativity and innovation to enhance nursing care;
- Participates in quality improvement initiatives;
- Collects data to monitor the quality of nursing practice;
- Contributes to efforts to improve healthcare efficiency;
- Provides critical review and evaluation of policies, procedures, and guidelines to improve the quality of care;
- Engages in formal and informal peer review processes of the interprofessional team;
- Collaborates with the interprofessional team to implement quality improvement plans and interventions;
- Documents nursing practice in a manner that supports quality and performance improvement initiatives; and
- Achieves or maintains neuroscience nursing certification.

ADDITIONAL COMPETENCIES FOR THE
GRADUATE-LEVEL PREPARED NEUROSCIENCE RN

In addition to the competencies of the neuroscience registered nurse, the graduate-level prepared neuroscience RN

- Uses data in system-level decision making;
- Analyzes trends in healthcare quality data, including examination of cultural influences and factors;
- Incorporates evidence into nursing practice to improve outcomes;
- Designs innovations to improve outcomes;
- Promotes a practice environment that supports evidence-based healthcare;
- Contributes to nursing and interprofessional knowledge through scientific inquiry;
- Encourages professional or specialty certification;
- Engages in development, implementation, evaluation, and revision of policies, procedures, and guidelines to improve healthcare quality;
- Designs quality improvement studies, research initiatives, and programs to improve health outcomes in diverse settings;
- Provides leadership in the design and implementation of quality improvement initiatives;
- Promotes compliance with internal and external regulatory requirements;
- Uses data and information in system-level decision-making;
- Influences the organizational system to improve outcomes; and
- Encourages professional or specialty certification.

ADDITIONAL COMPETENCIES FOR THE NEUROSCIENCE APRN

In addition to the competencies of the neuroscience nurse, the neuroscience APRN

- Engages in comparison evaluations of the effectiveness and efficacy of diagnostic tests, clinical procedures and therapies, and

treatment plans in partnership with healthcare consumers to
optimize health and healthcare quality;

- Applies knowledge obtained from advanced preparation, as well
  as current research and evidence-based information, to clinical
  decision-making at the point of care to achieve optimal health
  outcomes; and
- Uses available benchmarks as a means to evaluate practice at the
  individual, departmental, or organizational level.

Standard 16. Professional Practice Evaluation

The neuroscience nurse evaluates one's own and others' nursing practice.

COMPETENCIES

The neuroscience nurse

- Engages in self-reflection and self-evaluation of nursing practice
  on a regular basis, identifying areas of strength as well as areas in
  which professional growth would be beneficial;
- Adheres to professional practice guidance as specified in the
  Neuroscience Nursing: Scope and Standards of Practice and the
  Code of Ethics for Nurses with Interpretive Statements;
- Ensures that nursing practice is consistent with regulatory
  requirements pertaining to licensure, relevant laws, statutes,
  rules, and regulations while considering social determinants of
  health, diversity, equity and inclusion;
- Influences organizational policies and procedures to promote
  interprofessional evidence-based practice;
- Provides evidence to support practice decisions and actions as
  part of the evaluation process;
- Seeks feedback regarding one's own practice from healthcare
  consumers, peers, colleagues, supervisors, and others;
- Provides peers and others with constructive formal and informal
  feedback regarding their practice or role performance;

- Takes action to achieve learning needs and goals identified during the evaluation process by incorporating feedback received from consumers, peers, colleagues, supervisors, and others; and
- Documents the evaluative process, strategies used, and next steps to enhance one's own practice.

ADDITIONAL COMPETENCIES FOR THE GRADUATE-LEVEL PREPARED NEUROSCIENCE RN

In addition to the competencies of the neuroscience nurse, the graduate-level prepared neuroscience RN

- Disseminates best practices through activities such as presentations, publications, and consultations;
- Demonstrates leadership in evaluating practice to improve healthcare outcomes and quality of life;
- Mentors nurses to fulfill their professional role and responsibilities within their area of expertise;
- Volunteers and holds leadership positions in professional and specialty practice organizations;
- Influences development of evaluation standards and guidelines in their area of expertise; and
- Leads implementation and translation of evidence-based standards and guidelines into practice.

ADDITIONAL COMPETENCIES FOR THE NEUROSCIENCE APRN

In addition to the competencies of the neuroscience nurse and graduate-level prepared neuroscience RN, the neuroscience APRN

- Promotes and supports the development of advanced practice standards and guidelines in their area of expertise, and
- Evaluates professional practice data and benchmarks to enhance their own and other's practice.

Standard 17. Resource Stewardship

The neuroscience nurse utilizes appropriate resources to plan, provide, and sustain evidence-based nursing services that are safe, effective, equitable, financially responsible, and judiciously used.

COMPETENCIES

The neuroscience nurse

- Partners with the healthcare consumer and other stakeholders to identify care needs and necessary resources to achieve desired outcomes;
- Collaborates with the healthcare consumer and other stakeholders to assess costs, availability, risks, and benefits in decisions about care;
- Assists the healthcare consumer in identifying and securing appropriate resources to address needs across the healthcare continuum;
- Identifies impact of resource allocation on the potential for harm, task complexity, and desired outcomes;
- Advocates for equitable resources, including technology, that support and enhance nursing practice and health outcomes;
- Integrates connected health technologies, including telehealth and mobile options, into practice to promote positive interactions between healthcare consumers and care providers;
- Uses organizational and community resources to implement interprofessional plans; and
- Addresses discriminatory healthcare practices and the adverse impact on resource allocation.

ADDITIONAL COMPETENCIES FOR THE GRADUATE-LEVEL PREPARED NEUROSCIENCE RN, INCLUDING THE NEUROSCIENCE APRN

In addition to the competencies of the neuroscience nurse, the graduate-level prepared neuroscience RN, including the neuroscience APRN

- Employs epidemiologic modeling to assess and assist in the allocation of healthcare resources when limited or scarce;
- Creates processes that address cost-effectiveness, cost-benefits, and efficiency factors associated with nursing care;
- Addresses disparities in resource allocation and campaigns for equity and inclusion regardless of socioeconomic status;
- Designs collaborative and innovative strategies to effectively use resources and assign personnel in ways that maintain quality and reduce waste;
- Collaborates with interprofessional teams to optimize resources while considering cost to improve healthcare consumer outcomes;
- Assumes complex and advanced leadership roles to initiate and guide resource allocation based on evidence; and
- Serves as an expert to influence healthcare resource allocation policy.

Standard 18. Environmental Health

The neuroscience nurse practices in a manner that advances environmental safety and health.

COMPETENCIES

The neuroscience nurse

- Creates a safe and healthy workplace and professional practice environment;
- Fosters a professional environment that does not tolerate abusive, destructive, and oppressive behaviors for individuals, staff, and family units;
- Promotes evidence-based practices to create a psychologically and physically safe environment;
- Assesses the environment to identify and address risk factors that are associated with social determinants of health (see Standard 1);
- Reduces environmental health risks to self, colleagues, and healthcare consumers, and the world;

- Applies environmental health concepts in practice;
- Communicates information about environmental health risks and exposure reduction strategies;
- Advocates for the safe, judicious implementation of environmental health practice in communities where they work and live;
- Incorporates technologies to promote safe practice environments;
- Uses products or treatments consistent with evidence-based practice to reduce environmental threats and hazards;
- Examines how the healthcare consumer's biography affects their biology, resultant health issues, and the ecosystem;
- Analyzes the impacts of social, political, and economic influences on the human health experience and global environment;
- Advances environmental concerns and complaints through advocacy and appropriate reporting mechanisms; and
- Promotes sustainable global environmental health policies and conditions that focus on prevention of hazards to people and the natural environment.

ADDITIONAL COMPETENCIES FOR THE GRADUATE-LEVEL PREPARED NEUROSCIENCE RN, INCLUDING THE NEUROSCIENCE APRN

In addition to the competencies of the neuroscience nurse, the graduate-level prepared neuroscience RN, including the neuroscience APRN

- Designs research and evidence-based practice connections between the environment, its conditions, and health status, and
- Creates partnerships and uses data to develop policy, recommendations, and programs that promote sustainable global environmental health policies and conditions that focus on prevention of hazards to people and the natural environment.

Glossary

Acculturation. The process by which an individual or group from one culture learns how to take on many of the behaviors, values, and ways of living of another culture. Few cultures become 100% acculturated to another cultural way of life. Cultures tend to be selective in what they choose to change and retain (Leininger, 1995, pp. 72-73).

Advanced practice registered nurse (APRN). A subset of graduate-level prepared registered nurses who has completed an accredited graduate-level education preparing the nurse for special licensure and practice for one of four APRN roles: certified registered nurse anesthetist (CRNA), certified nurse-midwife (CNM), clinical nurse specialist (CNS), or certified nurse practitioner (CNP) (ANA, 2021, p. 109). Neuroscience APRN roles might include CRNA, CNS, or CNP.

Assessment. A systematic dynamic process by which the registered nurse, through interactions with the patient, family, groups, communities, populations, and healthcare providers, collects and analyses data. Assessment may include the following dimensions: physical, psychological, social-cultural, spiritual, cognitive, functional, developmental, economic, and lifestyle.

Autonomy. The capacity of a nurse to determine their own actions through independent choice, including demonstration of competence, within the full scope of nursing practice.

Caregiver. A person who provides direct care for another, such as a child, dependent adult, the disabled, or chronically ill (ANA, 2015).

Caring. The moral ideal of nursing consists of human-to-human attempts to protect, enhance, and preserve humanity and human dignity, integrity, and wholeness by assisting a person to find meaning in illness, suffering, pain, and existence (Watson, 2012).

Competence. Performing successfully at an expected level (ANA, 2014).

Competency. An expected level of performance that integrates knowledge, skills, human functioning, and judgment (ANA, 2014).

Graduate-level prepared registered nurse (RN). RNs who are prepared at the master's or doctoral level; have advanced knowledge, skills, abilities and judgement; function in an advanced level as designated by elements of the nurses' role; and are not required to have additional regulatory oversight (ANA, 2021, p. 112).

Healthcare. The prevention, treatment, and management of illness; the preservation of mental and physical well-being; and the promotion of health through the services offered by a healthcare provider or health professional.

Healthcare provider. A person licensed to provide care to individuals, including diagnosis and treatment of acute and chronic health problems.

Judgment. A characteristic of nursing competence that includes critical thinking, problem-solving, ethical reasoning, and decision-making.

Knowledge. A characteristic of nursing competence that encompasses thinking, understanding of science and humanities, professional standards of practice, and insights gained from practical experiences, personal capabilities, and leadership performance.

Liaison. A person whose function it is to maintain communication between or among individuals and an organization, parts of an organization, or between two or more organizations acting together for a common purpose.

Nursing. Integrates the art and science of caring and focuses on the protection, promotion, and optimization of health and human functioning, prevention of illness and injury, and alleviation of suffering through compassionate presence. Nursing is the diagnosis and treatment of human responses, and advocacy in the care of individuals, families, groups, communities, and populations in recognition of the connection of all humanity (ANA, 2021, p. 1).

Nursing process. A critical-thinking model used by nurses that is represented as the integration of the singular, concurrent, iterative actions of the six components of assessment, diagnosis, identification of outcomes, planning, implementation, and evaluation (ANA, 2021, p. 113). The nursing process encompasses all significant actions taken by RNs and forms the foundation of the neuroscience nurse's decision-making.

Population. Includes aggregates, persons with identified similarities, and communities.

Registered nurse (RN). An individual registered or licensed by a state, commonwealth, territory, government, or other regulatory body to practice under this title.

Skills. A characteristic of nursing competence that includes psychomotor, communication, interpersonal, and diagnostic abilities.

Standards. Authoritative statements of the duties that all RNs, regardless of role, population, or specialty, are expected to perform.

System. Any group of interacting, interrelated, or interdependent elements forming a complex whole.

References

American Association of Colleges of Nursing (AACN). (1998). *Certification and regulation of advanced practice nurse (AACN Position Statement).* Retrieved from www.aacn.nche.edu/Publications/positions/cereg.htm.

American Association of Neuroscience Nurses (AANN). (2015). *A position statement on the value of certification in neuroscience nursing.* Retrieved from https://aann.org/uploads/about/AANN_Position_Statement_on_the_Value_of_Certification.pdf

AANN. (2012). Care of the patient with intracranial pressure monitoring/external ventricular drainage or lumbar drainage. *AANN Clinical Practice Guideline Series.* Chicago, IL: Author.

AANN. (2014). Care of the adult patient with a brain tumor. *AANN Clinical Practice Guideline Series.* Chicago IL: Author.

AANN. (2021). Mobilization of the patient after neurological insult. *AANN Clinical Practice Guideline Series.* Chicago IL: Author.

American Nurses Association (ANA). (2015). *Code of ethics for nurses with interpretive statements.* Silver Spring, MD: Nursesbooks.org

ANA. (2014). *Professional role competence* (Position Statement). Silver Spring, MD: Author.

ANA. (2021). *Nursing: Scope and standards of practice* (4th ed.). Silver Spring, MD: Nursesbooks.org.

ANA. (2010). *Nursing's social policy statement: The essence of the profession.* Silver Spring, MD: Nursesbooks.org.

ANA. (2023). *Neurovascular nursing: Scope and standards of practice.* Silver Spring, MD: Nursesbooks.org.

American Nurses Credentialing Center (ANCC). (2014). Magnet model. Retrieved from https://www.nursingworld.org/organizational-programs/magnet/magnet-model/

ANCC. (2023). Magnet application manual updates and FAQs. Retrieved from https://www.nursingworld.org/organizational-programs/magnet/magnet-manual-updates-and-faqs/

Advanced Practice Registered Nurse Joint Dialogue Group (APRN JDG). (2008). *Consensus Model for APRN Regulation: Licensure, Accreditation, Certification and Education.* Retrieved from https://www.nursingworld.org/~4aa7d9/globalassets/certification/aprn_consensus_model_report_7-7-08.pdf

Aycock, D. M., Clark, P. C., Hayat, M. J., Salazar, L. F., & Eriksen, M. P. (2023). Stroke Counseling intervention for young adult African Americans: A randomized controlled trial. *Nursing Research, 72*(2), 83–92. https://doi.org/10.1097/NNR.0000000000000633

Bautista, C., Hinkle, J. L., Alexander, S., Hundt, B., & Rhudy, L. (2022). A Delphi study to establish research priorities for neuroscience nursing. *The Journal of Neuroscience Nursing: Journal of the American Association of Neuroscience Nurses, 54*(2), 74–79. Retrieved from https://doi.org/10.1097/JNN.0000000000000637

Buxton, K., Morgan, A. & Rogers, J. (2017). Nurse practitioner lead pediatric baclofen pump program: Impact on safety and quality of care. *Journal of Neuroscience Nursing, 49*(5), 325–329. Retrieved from https://doi.org/10.1097/JNN.0000000000000310

Drollinger, L., & Prasun, M. A. (2023). Bundled approach to improve inpatient stroke recognition and time to treatment. *The Journal of Neuroscience Nursing, 55*(1), 18–23. Retrieved from https://doi.org/10.1097/JNN.0000000000000685

Gallagher-Lepak, S., & Kubsch, S. (2009). Transpersonal caring: A nursing practice guideline. *Holistic Nursing Practice, 23*, 171–182.

Helms, A. M., Yang, H., Karamchandani, R. R., Williams, L., Singh, S., DeFilipp, G. J., & Asimos, A. W. (2023). A telestroke nurse and neuroradiologist model for extended window code stroke triage. *The Journal of Neuroscience Nursing, 55*(3), 74–79. Retrieved from https://doi.org/10.1097/JNN.0000000000000700

Hickey, J., Duffy, L. V., Hinkle, J. L., Prendergast, V., Rhudy, L. M., Sullivan, C., & Villanueva, N. E. (2019). Scholarship in neuroscience nursing. *Journal of Neuroscience Nursing, 51*(5), 243–248. Retrieved from https://doi.org/10.1097/JNN.0000000000000465

Hickey, J. V. & Strayer, A.L. (2020). *The clinical practice of neurological & neurosurgical nursing* (8th ed.). Philadelphia, PA: Lippincott Williams & Wilkins.

Hinkle, J. L., Sullivan, C., Villanueva, N., & Hickey, J.C. (2012). Integrating the Institute of Medicine future of nursing report into the American Association of Neuroscience Nurses strategic plan. *Journal of Neuroscience Nursing, 44*(3), 164–167. Retrieved from https://doi.org/10.1097/JNN.0b013e31825106a2

Holleman, J., Johnson, A., & Frim, D. (2010). The impact of a 'resident replacement' nurse practitioner on an academic pediatric neurosurgical service. *Pediatric Neurosurgery, 46*(3), 177–181.

Institute of Medicine (IOM). (2009). *Forum on the future of nursing: Acute care* (pp. 28–33). Washington, DC: National Academies Press. Retrieved from http://www.nap.edu/catalog.php?record_id=12855

IOM. (2004). *Keeping patients safe: Transforming the work environment of nurses.* Washington, DC: National Academies Press.

Jaffa, J.L., Dufault, M., & Lavin, M. (2017). An interprofessional approach to amyotrophic lateral sclerosis care. *Journal of Neuroscience Nursing, 49*(5), 319–323. Retrieved from https://doi.org/10.1097/JNN.0000000000000309

Leininger, M. (1995). *Transcultural nursing. Concepts, theories, research & practices* (2nd ed.). New York, NY: McGraw-Hill Education.

Madden, L.K., Hundley, L., Summers, D., Villanueva, N., & Walter, S.M. (2017). Assessing the American Association of Neuroscience Nurses' progress on the Institute of Medicine report. *Journal of Neuroscience Nursing, 49*(3), 146–150. Retrieved from https://doi.org/10.1097/JNN.0000000000000285

Mills, N., Bachmann, M.O., Campbell, R., Hine, I., & McGowan, M. (1999). Effect of a primary care based epilepsy specialist nurse service on quality of care from the patients' perspective: Results at two-years follow-up. *Seizure, 8*(5), 291–296.

Mitchell, E., Reynolds, S. S., Mower-Wade, D., Raser-Schramm, J., & Granger, B. B. (2022). Implementation of an advanced practice registered nurse-led clinic to improve follow-up care for post-ischemic stroke patients. *The Journal of Neuroscience Nursing: Journal of the American Association of Neuroscience Nurses, 54*(5), 193–198. Retrieved from https://doi.org/10.1097/JNN.0000000000000670

Moyer, M., Hinkle, J. L., & Mendez, J. D. (2021). An integrative review: Early mobilization of patients with external ventriculostomy drains in the neurological intensive care unit. *Journal of Neuroscience Nursing, 53*(5), 220. Retrieved from https://doi.org/10.1097/JNN.0000000000000609

National Academy of Medicine. (2021). *The future of nursing 2020–2030: Charting a path to achieve health equity.* Retrieved from https://www.nam.edu/wp-content/uploads/2022/01/nursing.jpg

Olson, D. (2017). Defining neuroscience nursing. *Journal of Neuroscience Nursing, 49*(6), 332. Retrieved from https://doi.org/10.1097/JNN.0000000000000278

Pituch, K. J., Simon, N., Weaver, M. S., & Lindley, L. C. (2022). Preparing a pediatric palliative care program for sustainable support: A practice reflection. *The Journal of Neuroscience Nursing, 54*(5), 199–200. Retrieved from https://doi.org/10.1097/JNN.0000000000000659

Prendergast, V., Elmasry, S., Juhl, N. A., & Chapple, K. M. (2023). Resilience room use and its effect on distress among nurses and allied staff. *The Journal of Neuroscience Nursing, 55*(3), 80–85.

Stewart-Amidei, C., & Kunkel, J.A. (Eds.). (2000). *AANN's neuroscience nursing: human responses to neurologic dysfunction* (2nd ed.). Philadelphia, PA: Saunders.

Stewart-Amidei, C., Villanueva, N., Schwartz, R.R., Delemos, C., West, T., Tocco, S., et al. (2010). American Association of Neuroscience Nurses scope and standards of practice for neuroscience advanced practice nurses. *Journal of Neuroscience Nursing, 42*(3), E1–E8.

Villanueva, N., Blank-Reid, C., Stewart-Amidei, C., Cartwright, C., Haymore, & Jones, R.W. (2008). The role of the advanced practice nurse in neuroscience nursing. *Journal of Neuroscience Nursing, 40*(2), 119–124.

Villaruel, A. M., & James, R. (2022). Preventing the spread of misinformation: A role for all nurses. *American Nurse Today, 17*(2), 22.

Watson, J. (2012). *Human caring science: A theory of nursing* (2nd ed.). Sudbury, MA: Jones and Bartlett Learning.

Webb, D. (2000). Scope of neuroscience nursing. In C. Stewart-Amidei & J.A. Kunkel (Eds.), *AANN's neuroscience nursing: Human responses to neurologic dysfunction* (2nd ed., pp. 3-11). Philadelphia, PA: Saunders.

Yeager, S. (2009). The neuroscience acute care nurse practitioner: Role development, implementation, and improvement. *Critical Care Nursing Clinics of North America, 21*(4), 561–593. Retrieved from https://doi.org/10.1016/j.ccell.2009.07.008

Yeager, S., Shaw, K.D., Casavant, J., & Burns, S.M. (2006). An acute care nurse practitioner model of care for neurosurgical patients. *Critical Care Nurse, 26*(6), 57–64.

Index